Integrated Clinical Science

Psychiatry

Integrated Clinical Science

Other titles:

Cardiovascular Disease
Professor JR Hampton

Haematology
JC Cawley

Nephro-urology
Professor AW Asscher
Professor DB Moffat

Respiratory Disease
GM Sterling

Musculoskeletal Disease
Professor V Wright and
Professor R Dickson

Gastroenterology
P Jones, P Brunt,
NAG Mowat

Neurology
RW Ross Russell

Endocrinology
Professor CRW Edwards

Projected:

Human Health and the Environment

Reproduction and Development

Integrated Clinical Science

Psychiatry

Edited by

J.L.Gibbons MD, FRCP, FRCPsych

Professor of Psychiatry, University of Southampton
Honorary Consultant Psychiatrist,
Southampton District Health Authority

Series Editor

George P. McNicol, MD, PhD, FRCP
(Lond, Edin, Glasg), FRCPath, Hon FACP

Principal and Vice Chancellor, University of Aberdeen. Lately Professor of
Medicine, The University of Leeds, and Head, The University Department
of Medicine, The General Infirmary, Leeds

William Heinemann Medical Books Ltd
London

ISBN 0-433-16605-3

© 1983 William Heinemann Medical Books Ltd,
23 Bedford Square,
London WC1B 3HH

First published 1983
Reprinted 1985

Printed and bound in Great Britain by the
Alden Press, Oxford

Contents

Preface

It is clearly desirable on educational grounds to adopt and teach a rational approach to the management of patients, whereby the basic scientific knowledge, the applied science and the art of clinical practice are brought together in an integrated way. Progress has been made in this direction, but after twenty-five years of good intentions, teaching in many medical schools is still split up into three large compartments, preclinical, paraclinical and clinical, and further subdivided on a disciplinary basis. Lip-service is paid to integration, but what emerges is often at best a coordinated rather than an integrated curriculum. Publication of the INTEGRATED CLINICAL SCIENCE series reflects the need felt in many quarters for a truly integrated textbook series, and is also intended as a stimulus to further reform of the curriculum.

The complete series will cover the core of clinical teaching, each volume dealing with a particular body system. Revision material in the basic sciences of anatomy, physiology, biochemistry and pharmacology is presented at the level of detail appropriate for Final MB examinations, and subsequently for rational clinical practice. Integration between the volumes ensures complete and consistent coverage of these areas, and similar principles govern the treatment of the clinical disciplines of medicine, surgery, pathology, microbiology, immunology and epidemiology.

The series is planned to give a reasoned rather than a purely descriptive account of clinical practice and its scientific basis. Clinical manifestations are described in relation to the disorders of structure and function which occur in a disease process. Illustrations are used extensively, and are an integral part of the text.

The editors for each volume, well-known as authorities and teachers in their fields, have been recruited from medical schools throughout the UK. Chapter contributors are even more widely distributed, and coordination between the volumes has been supervised by a distinguished team of specialists.

Each volume in the series represents a component in an overall plan of approach to clinical teaching. It is intended, nevertheless, that every volume should be self-sufficient as an account of its own subject area, and all the basic and clinical science with which an undergraduate could reasonably be expected to be familiar is presented in the appropriate volume. It is expected that, whether studied individually or as a series, the volumes of INTEGRATED CLINICAL SCIENCE will meet a major need, assisting teachers and students to adopt a more rational and holistic approach in learning to care for the sick.

George P. McNicol
Series Editor

Contributors

Brian Barraclough
Senior Lecturer in Psychiatry
University of Southampton
and Honorary Consultant Psychiatrist
Royal South Hants Hospital
Southampton

John Brunning
Consultant Psychiatrist
St James Hospital
Portsmouth
and Honorary Clinical Teacher in Psychiatry
University of Southampton

Guy Edwards
Consultant Psychiatrist
Royal South Hants Hospital
Southampton
and Honorary Clinical Teacher in Psychiatry
University of Southampton

Robert Fieldsend
Consultant Psychiatrist
St John's Hospital
Stone Aylesbury
Bucks

Professor James Gibbons
Professor of Psychiatry
University of Southampton
and Honorary Consultant Psychiatrist
Southampton District Health Authority

Keith Hawton
Clinical Tutor
Department of Psychiatry
Oxford University
Warneford Hospital
Oxford

Jennifer Hughes
Senior Research Fellow in Psychiatry
University of Southampton
and Honorary Consultant Psychiatrist
Royal South Hants Hospital
Southampton

Robin Jacoby
Consultant Psychiatrist
Maudsley Hospital
London

George Szmukler
Senior Lecturer in Psychiatry
Institute of Psychiatry
and Honorary Consultant
Maudsley Hospital
London

Pamela Taylor
Senior Lecturer in Forensic Psychiatry
Institute of Psychiatry
and Honorary Consultant
Maudsley Hospital
London

Carol Trotter
Consultant Psychiatrist (Psychogeriatrics)
St James Hospital
Portsmouth
and Honorary Clinical Teacher in Psychiatry
University of Southampton

Peter Tyrer
Consultant Psychiatrist
Mapperley Hospital
Nottingham

Advisory Editors

Professor A Stuart Douglas
Department of Medicine, University of Aberdeen

Pathology: Professor CC Bird
Institute of Pathology
University of Leeds

Anatomy: Professor RL Holmes
Department of Anatomy
University of Leeds

Physiology: Professor PH Fentem
Department of Physiology and
Pharmacology
Nottingham University

Pharmacology: Professor AM Breckenridge
Department of Clinical
Pharmacology
Liverpool University

Biochemistry: Dr RM Denton
Reader in Biochemistry
University of Bristol

Introduction

This book has been written for medical students. It aims to provide enough theoretical background for the student to understand the classification of psychiatric disorders (Chapter 1), and then to show how the psychiatric assessment of an individual patient is carried out, at the same time illustrating many important psychiatric symptoms (Chapter 2). An account of the classical psychiatric syndromes follows (Chapters 3–6). Here particular attention is paid to organic disorders and to minor psychiatric disorders (the neuroses), both of which are more likely to present to clinicians other than psychiatrists. The psychiatric effects of primarily physical illnesses are also considered. The care of the elderly mentally ill is becoming increasingly important as our population ages, justifying separate consideration of the influence of ageing on the incidence and the clinical manifestations of psychiatric disorders (Chapter 7).

The book then deals with four topics that are of interest to many other clinicians besides psychiatrists. Deliberate self harm ('attempted suicide') is a major problem for casualty departments and for departments of general medicine (Chapter 8), while the effects of excessive alcohol intake are important for almost all clinicians (Chapter 9). In order to illustrate the modern 'psychosomatic' approach, Chapter 10 discusses the psychological aspects of feeding disorders. This section of the book ends with an account of psychosexual disorders, a field in which there have been important recent advances in our knowledge of aetiology and treatment (Chapter 11).

Chapters 12 and 13, dealing with the general principles of psychological and physical methods of treatment in psychiatry, constitute brief overviews of their respective topics. They should be read in conjunction with the sections on treatment of specific disorders in other chapters.

In Chapter 14 the student will find a rather fuller than usual account of the law relating to the mentally ill in England and Wales. This is to help the student appreciate the difficulties in protecting the patient and society on the one hand, and in preserving the liberty of the subject on the other. Mental health law has become an important topic of public debate and in 1983 a new Mental Health Act has reached the statute book. Chapter 14 ensures that the student is adequately informed about this whole important area. Finally Chapter 15 deals with another topic of public concern and misapprehension, the relationship between crime and mental disorder.

1

Nature and Classification of Psychiatric Disorder

Psychiatry is the branch of medicine which is concerned with the study and treatment of mental disorders – illness and other abnormalities that present with predominantly (or entirely) psychological symptoms and/or disturbances of behaviour.

HISTORICAL INTRODUCTION

Madness has always been recognised. In the past it has sometimes been attributed to illness (as by the physicians of classical Greece), sometimes to divine or diabolical influence (as by the poets of classical Greece and the physicians of medieval Europe). Systematic study of mental illness only became possible when sufficiently large numbers of patients could be studied by trained observers over long periods of time in humane conditions. This opportunity only became available at the end of the eighteenth century, a time of revolutionary ideas and of the spirit of 'liberty, equality and brotherhood'. It is not surprising that the first studies were carried out in revolutionary France. Further work was carried out in France and afterwards in Germany during the nineteenth century.

These early French and German investigators – like many psychiatric research workers today –

used what John Wing has called 'disease theories' in their search for disease entities with a uniform symptomatology, course, outcome and (it was hoped) aetiology. The first stage in the development of a disease theory is the recognition of a cluster of symptoms – a syndrome – which is reasonably stable over time and which is not characterised only by social phenomena such as deviant behaviour. The next stage is the discovery of underlying biological abnormalities, which often comprise disturbed homeostatic mechanisms. It soon became clear that some mentally ill patients were ill because of brain disease, or because of disease or some other abnormality elsewhere in the body that severely compromised brain function; these patients were suffering from organic psychiatric disorders. In the remaining patients no relevant pathological changes could be demonstrated post-mortem in the brain or elsewhere in the body. These were therefore said to suffer from 'functional' mental disorder.

The nineteenth-century psychiatrists were mainly concerned with severely ill patients who suffered from organic or functional psychoses. Patients suffering from less severe mental disorders – the neuroses – were investigated particularly by neurologists and we owe our first good descriptions of neurotic syndromes to French- and German-speaking neurologists such as Charcot and Freud.

CLASSIFICATION OF PSYCHIATRIC DISORDERS

As a result of the French and German clinical studies mentioned already, we can construct the simple scheme of classification shown in Fig. 1.1.

The term psychosis has two meanings. Strictly it is a descriptive term that refers to the disorders classified in Categories I and II of the figure. When one of these disorders is fully developed, the patient's symptoms and behaviour would suggest insanity to lay people; the patient may announce totally irrational beliefs, listen to non-existent voices, behave in a strange, bewildering and unaccountable way and have no awareness (insight) of his morbid state. Not all cases of these disorders – organic and functional psychoses – are so severe, however, and some patients are aware that they are ill. Psychosis – and especially its adjectival form, psychotic – is also used to describe a particularly severe degree of mental disorder, when the patient is deluded, hallucinated, or otherwise out of touch with reality. In the neuroses such 'psychotic' features are not seen; the patient's personality is not grossly distorted and contact with reality is maintained. Neurotic subjects would not be regarded by lay people as 'insane', but possibly as 'nervous'.

The student should note that the classification illustrated in Fig. 1.1 is a hierarchical one, with higher categories taking diagnostic precedence over lower categories. In consequence, functional psychosis can only be diagnosed if features of organic psychoses are absent. In Britain and Western Europe, at least, the presence of definite and persistent schizophrenic features requires a diagnosis of schizophrenia even if characteristic features of affective psychosis (in which the principal feature is elevation or depression of mood) are also present. Neurotic symptoms are almost always present in both organic and functional psychoses, but the diagnosis of neurosis is made only when a neurotic syndrome occurs in

the absence of clear features of either organic or functional psychosis (Categories I and II, Fig. 1.1).

Organic Syndromes

These are described in Chapter 3. As in psychiatric practice generally, the diagnosis of an organic psychosyndrome (clouding of consciousness in the acute disorder, impairment of memory and intelligence in the chronic) depends on the recognition of the cluster of typical clinical features; it may sometimes be confirmed by specialised psychological tests. The nature of the underlying physical cause may be revealed by the history (e.g. alcohol withdrawal leading to delirium tremens; a family history of dementia and involuntary movements in a case of Huntington's chorea) or may require physical methods of investigation (e.g. serology in syphilitic general paresis; neuroradiology in cerebral tumour). The student must remember, however, that psychosocial factors may be very important for patients suffering from organic disorders. Reference to Chapter 7 will illustrate this statement.

Functional Psychoses

In this general category we owe the distinction between the two broad groups of schizophrenic (Chapter 4) and affective (Chapter 5) psychoses to early German psychiatrists, particularly Emil Kraepelin. They were concerned not only with the recognition of syndromes, but also with the course of the illnesses, with the longitudinal study of numerous individual patients over many years. A more recent research worker has suggested that long-term follow-up is the psychiatric equivalent of autopsy in the study of physical disease.

One can argue that some aspects of psychotic experience are different in kind from normal experience. Thus, some patients suffering from depressive psychosis say that their depressed

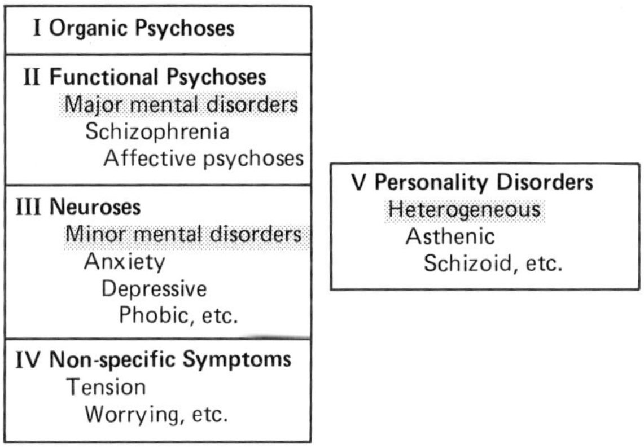

```
┌─────────────────────────────────┐
│ I Organic Psychoses             │
├─────────────────────────────────┤
│ II Functional Psychoses         │
│    Major mental disorders       │
│    Schizophrenia                │
│    Affective psychoses          │        ┌──────────────────────────┐
├─────────────────────────────────┤        │ V Personality Disorders  │
│ III Neuroses                    │        │    Heterogeneous         │
│     Minor mental disorders      │        │    Asthenic              │
│     Anxiety                     │        │      Schizoid, etc.      │
│     Depressive                  │        └──────────────────────────┘
│       Phobic, etc.              │
├─────────────────────────────────┤
│ IV Non-specific Symptoms        │
│    Tension                      │
│      Worrying, etc.             │
└─────────────────────────────────┘
```

Fig. 1.1. *A simple hierarchical classification of psychiatric disorders.*

mood has a quality distinct from that of ordinary unhappiness. Schizophrenics have experiences of a kind that the rest of humanity never has (outside of dreams). At all events most psychiatrists feel justified in applying disease theories to the functional psychoses, perhaps believing that subtle neurochemical abnormalities underly the principal symptoms, while recognising that psychosocial events often exert an important influence on their course and outcome. Dissenting views are briefly discussed below.

Neuroses

These disorders (Chapter 6) are much commoner than the functional psychoses; only a small and highly selected sample of neurotic patients reaches the psychiatrist. Several specific forms of neurosis occur (e.g. phobic and obsessional neuroses), but the vast majority of neurotic patients suffer from depression or anxiety or both. Neurosis can generally be regarded as only quantitatively different from normal; neurotic anxiety differs from healthy anxiety only in degree. That does not mean that it is inappropriate to formulate disease theories about the neuroses. There is, after all, no clear dividing line between normal and raised blood pressure or fasting blood sugar.

Neurotic symptoms often mimic physical illness (for example, the epigastric unrest of anxiety misinterpreted by the patient, and perhaps also by the doctor, as dyspepsia or pain) and they may complicate physical illness (for example, anxiety or depression exacerbating the disability due to chronic bronchitis or rheumatoid arthritis). Consequently all clinicians can expect to see neurotic patients quite often. Knowledge of the neuroses is therefore necessary in all forms of clinical practice, most of all in primary medical care.

Other Disorders

The term personality disorder (Chapter 6) is applied to a heterogeneous group of people who suffer, or cause society to suffer, because of their abnormal personality traits. Disease theories seem quite inappropriate in this field. The same is true of non-specific complaints such as worrying and tension, which are best regarded as part of the human condition.

A number of other disorders, which often lead to referral to a psychiatric clinic, do not fit easily into the simplified schema of Fig. 1.1. They include alcohol and drug abuse, psychosexual disorders, most cases of deliberate self-harm and anorexia nervosa.

Concepts of Mental Illness

Psychiatrists are often asked to see people whose behaviour has been so extreme that mental illness is suggested as the only possible explanation. We have already seen how a disease theory cannot be based purely on social or behavioural features. Aubrey Lewis, who played a major role in the development of academic psychiatry in Britain, argued that mental illness must involve the disturbance of individual psychological functions – he called them 'part-functions' – such as perception, memory, thinking or mood. Global behaviour disturbance, whether crime or eccentricity or simple nuisance, cannot be attributed to mental illness unless one or more of the part-functions is clearly disturbed.

Several influential critics of orthodox psychiatry, most of them in North America, have denied the existence of mental illness (by which they often seem to mean schizophrenia) altogether. According to one view, organic psychiatric disorders are illnesses because they are due to demonstrable physical disease or dysfunction, but they are physical rather than mental illnesses. All functional psychiatric disorders are problems of living which neither excuse the sufferer from the legal consequences of his actions nor warrant his detention if he has committed no crime. Another view regards mental illness as a convenient 'label' applied by the psychiatrist to forms of deviant behaviour that society will not tolerate. Once a person has been labelled as mentally ill, both his own and other people's perception of him and expectations of his future behaviour are changed and he behaves as a mentally ill person should. Labelling a person as mentally ill can, of course, have unfortunate consequences. A former resident of a psychiatric hospital, involved in a fracas in the street, may well find himself returned to hospital rather than detained in a police station. Nevertheless, it is difficult to see how labelling would induce in a person such strange and bewildering experiences as thought insertion or thought withdrawal in schizophrenia (p.35).

The ICD Classification

We attempt to classify psychiatric disorder for several reasons: to provide a structure to enable us to communicate with other clinicians, to provide statistics for service planners, to make epidemiological studies of psychiatric disorders possible, and so on. Many centres have their own private classifications, based on their own theoretical attitudes, but it is important to have a public classification which everyone can understand and which can be used for the international exchange of information. One such classification is provided by the ninth revision of the International Classification of Disease (ICD), produced under the auspices of the World Health Organisation. The psychiatric section contains a glossary, in which the disorders listed in the section are briefly described. The main psychiatric categories are listed in Table 1.1. Each is denoted by a three figure number; subcategories are denoted by a fourth digit. Thus, all forms of schizophrenia are coded under 295. Paranoid schizophrenia, for example, is 295.3. In the same way 300 includes the neuroses, with anxiety states as 300.0, phobic states 300.2 and so on.

AETIOLOGY OF PSYCHIATRIC DISORDERS

There are various theoretical approaches which attempt to offer a comprehensive explanation for some or all psychiatric disorders. Psychoanalytic theory explains all psychiatric disorders in psychological terms, although the basic instinctual forces have a biological origin. Behavioural psychology regards the symptoms of functional disorders (and the disorders amount to no more than the sum of

Table 1.1

Principal Categories of the ICD Classification of Psychiatric Disorders

Organic psychoses (290–4)
290   Senile and presenile dementia
291   Alcoholic psychoses, e.g. 291.0 – Delirium tremens
292   Drug-induced psychoses
293   Transient organic psychoses, e.g. 293.0 – Acute delirium

Other Psychoses (295–9)
295   Schizophrenia, e.g. 295.3 – Paranoid schizophrenia
296   Affective psychoses, e.g. 296.1 – Unipolar depressive psychosis
                                   296.3 – Bipolar depressive psychosis
297   Paranoid states

Neurotic Disorders, Personality Disorders, etc. (300–16)
300   Neuroses, e.g. 300.0 – Anxiety states
                     300.2 – Phobic states
                     300.4 – Neurotic depression
301   Personality disorders, e.g. 301.2 – Schizoid
                                  301.4 – Anankastic
                                  301.6 – Asthenic
                                  301.7 – Sociopathic
302   Sexual deviations and disorders
303   Alcohol dependence
304   Drug dependence
305   Non-dependent abuse of drugs (and alcohol)
307   Other special syndromes, e.g. 307.1 – Anorexia nervosa

the symptoms) as learned maladaptive responses, the product of the individual's unique experiences and the universal laws of learning. There may still be 'organic' psychiatrists who regard psychiatric symptoms as irrelevant epiphenomena of as-yet undiscovered brain diseases.

For the rest of us the aetiology of functional psychiatric disorders is uncertain and probably almost always multifactorial. There are few necessary causes in psychiatry; perhaps schizophrenia and manic-depressive illness can only develop in people with the appropriate genetic predisposition, the nature of which is unknown in both cases. One necessary cause is the *Treponema pallidum*, without which there can be no neurosyphilis. The early treatment of venereal disease with antibiotics has made neurosyphilis a rare cause of organic psychosis. Even when

untreated syphilis was common, only a minority of sufferers developed general paresis. Some of them quietly demented; others, before intellectual deterioration became very severe, showed a mixture of organic symptoms with manic, depressive or schizophrenic syndromes. Obviously factors other than the infecting micro-organism determined whether neurosyphilis occurred and what the presenting psychiatric symptoms were.

Predisposing Factors

It is reasonable to suppose that an increased liability to develop later psychiatric disorder may be due to genetic endowment, to early life experience or to interaction between the two. There is evidence for a strong genetic factor in the functional psychoses, a weaker one in the neuroses. Important life experience may be of a psychosocial kind (e.g. emotional deprivation), of a physical kind (malnutrition, minor brain damage), or there may be a psychological reaction to a physical disorder (prolonged stay in hospital in early childhood, sensitivity because of a physical handicap).

Often there appear to be two aspects of predisposition to later illness. One is the liability to develop a particular disorder, the other is vulnerability to particular forms of threatening life events in adulthood. One person develops symptoms after a bereavement, another after a career disappointment, another after the first experience of physical symptoms severe enough to raise the spectre of mortality.

Personality results from a combination of genetic influence and early rearing, and certain personalities are more likely to develop adult psychiatric disorder. Thus, anxiety-prone individuals are over-represented among neurotic patients, while people with some aspects of obsessional personality seem to have an increased risk of developing a depressive illness.

Personality may also have an effect on psychiatric illness by modifying the usual clinical picture. Patients who have always been suspicious and solitary may develop marked persecutory delusions, severe enough to suggest a diagnosis of a paranoid psychosis (p.40), during a major depressive episode. Similarly, an episode of anxiety or depression may present with striking obsessional symptoms in a patient with marked obsessional personality traits.

Precipitating Factors

Some functional psychiatric illnesses appear out of the blue; only an indefatigable searcher with preconceived notions can find any precipitant. Others occur in association with physical disease. Sometimes the psychiatric disorder can be best understood as a psychological reaction to the physical disorder (p.29), sometimes the causal link seems more direct, as when a schizophrenic syndrome complicates brain disease or excessive alcohol intake, or when a depressive syndrome complicates infectious mononucleosis, hypothyroidism or Cushing's syndrome. Such functional disorders, occurring in direct association with cerebral, endocrine or other physical disease, are sometimes known as 'symptomatic' psychoses or neuroses.

In the last 20 years there has been a great deal of work on the relationship between life events and the subsequent onset of psychiatric (and, indeed, of physical) illness. The earlier work had methodological weakness, but sounder recent work has produced strong, if not quite compelling, evidence that a threatening life event may precipitate an episode of acute schizophrenia within two or three weeks and may precipitate, and perhaps even cause, an episode of depression within the next nine months. The type of life event associated with depression is characteristically real or threatened loss. There is some evidence that events involving danger – events raising the possibility of unpleasant crisis in the future – may be associated with a subsequent episode of anxiety.

What appears to be the same life event may, of course, be threatening to one person but not to another. Loss of a job might be a shattering blow to self-esteem, or a welcome relief from unbearable responsibility.

Neural Basis of Psychiatric Disorders

Little is known about this topic. We know that lesions in certain areas of the brain can produce particular organic symptoms. For example, the amnestic syndrome is due to bilateral midbrain, thalamic or hippocampal lesions (p.22). In the case of the functional psychoses there is some evidence that certain neuronal systems may be involved – the mesolimbic dopaminergic system in schizophrenia and certain noradrenergic or serotoninergic neurones in depression. A great deal of work on the possible relationship between particular psychiatric syndromes and dysfunction in one or other cerebral hemisphere has left us still uncertain except for the tentative conclusion that in schizophrenia the neural disturbance begins in the left hemisphere.

2

The Approach to the Patient

THE GENERAL APPROACH

The aim of the psychiatric interview is to gather information about the past and present condition of the patient in order that a diagnosis and plan for treatment may be reached. In this respect it is similar to a general medical examination. The medical examination, however, is then augmented by further investigations, whereas the psychiatric examination is usually the only investigatory procedure available. The psychiatric interview is also a form of treatment, and the gathering of information must not be at the expense of providing a therapeutic experience for the patient. Feelings, as well as facts, must be elicited. Skill is required to obtain information without appearing to interrogate the patient, particularly as the nature of the patient's problems may render him unable to communicate with ease.

The first few minutes of contact with the patient set the scene for the interview. Valuable time may be wasted by an interviewer who adopts a hurried and tactless approach. When the patient enters the room it is courteous to stand up and greet him with a smile. The interviewer should introduce himself clearly and briefly explain the purpose of the interview. The way in which the room is arranged is also important. Many psychiatrists find that sitting behind a desk leads to a feeling of remoteness from the patient. A good compromise may be to sit beside the desk with the patient

sitting at right angles to the interviewer (Fig. 2.1). Patient and interviewer should be seated on chairs of the same height.

The interviewer now seeks to obtain enough information to come to some conclusions about the diagnosis, severity of illness and the likely prognosis after treatment. This must be done in a manner that puts the patient at ease. The mere recounting of the history can help the patient, who may gain considerable insight during the interview.

The form in which questions are put needs careful consideration. Wherever possible the

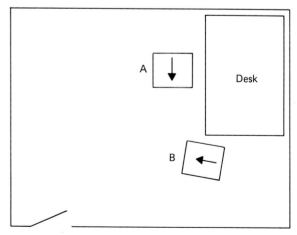

Fig. 2.1 *Suggested position of chairs. A—Interviewer, B—Patient.*

exploration of each aspect of the history should begin with an open ended question. An open ended question allows the patient to give an extended reply. For example, a useful open ended question with which to commence might be 'Can you tell me how you have been feeling recently?'. This question allows the patient to describe the presenting complaint and enables the interviewer to go on to ask more specific questions about the presenting complaint – the history of the presenting complaint (Fig. 2.2). More specific questions, for example, about mood, could again begin with an open ended question 'How have you been in your spirits recently?'. This is better than the use of a closed question such as 'Have you been depressed?'. A closed question invites a yes/no answer only. When a patient is reluctant to talk spontaneously about how he has been feeling, closed questions may be necessary. For example, a closed question with alternatives may be helpful 'Have you been feeling particularly happy, sad or just normal recently?'. Closed questions are also usually necessary to obtain accurate information about a symptom disclosed as a result of a series of open ended questions. Examples of open and closed questions to elucidate suicidal feelings are

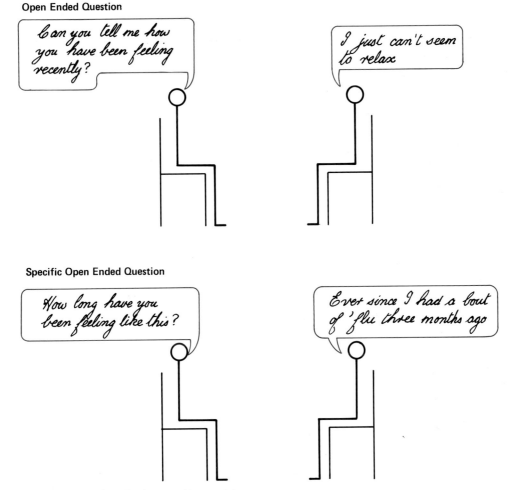

Open Ended Question

Can you tell me how you have been feeling recently?

I just can't seem to relax

Specific Open Ended Question

How long have you been feeling like this?

Ever since I had a bout of 'flu three months ago

Fig. 2.2 *The presenting complaint, leading into history of the presenting complaint.*

shown in Fig. 2.3; Fig. 2.4 shows examples of open and closed questions related to childhood.

Another way to obtain more information on a particular topic is to use checks (near repetitions in an interrogative tone of what the patient has just said). For example, the interviewer might ask 'How do you get on with your husband?'. The patient might reply 'We have our ups and downs'. The interviewer might then say 'You have ups and downs?'. This may encourage the patient to volunteer more information about the significance of the 'ups and downs'.

The recounting of past painful experiences may distress the patient. A skilled interviewer listens patiently and judges the tactful time to intervene with the next question, or encourages further disclosure of the painful subject by using sympathetic or reflective comments. Such comments can help and encourage the patient to share his painful feelings· and realise that the interviewer understands him and is not embarrassed by his tears. Examples of reflective comments in response to a patient who becomes tearful when recounting a past event might be 'That must have been very upsetting for you' or 'I wonder how that made you feel?'.

Patients with severe mental illness may be so withdrawn, distractible or muddled that a full history cannot be obtained. The interviewer must then decide how long to persevere with questioning and may need to be content with a very patchy history from the patient. Close friends or relatives may then help to fill in the gaps. On the whole it is better to obtain the patient's permission to talk to relatives, although with some psychotic patients with no insight this may not be possible. Remember, however, that relatives' opinions about the patient may be biased. It is wise to ask the relative how much of the information disclosed can be shared with the patient later, without undermining the patient's trust in his relative. It may be useful to conduct an interview with a relative or friend present. This way the patient is not left wondering what has been said 'behind his back'. In a joint interview it is important to ensure that the patient does not feel he is being talked about in his presence.

Taking of notes during an interview makes some patients feel uncomfortable. If the interviewer writes full notes, the amount of attention paid to the patient by eye-to-eye contact may be very small. With practice the interviewer can remember a surprising amount of the history and can avoid writing detailed notes until afterwards. It may be helpful to prepare headings on notepaper before the start of the interview.

Finally, the student who is attempting to learn how to interview patients must develop a self-scrutinising approach. This is best done with the help of videotape feedback. If this is not available, the use of audiotaped interviews may be almost as valuable. The patient's permission must be sought before any interview is taped and the contents of the tape erased when the learning exercise is completed.

THE HISTORY

The following is a description of the information that the interviewer might be expected to obtain, in the order in which the interview is eventually recorded. The actual questions asked may not follow this order and must be tailored to suit the individual patient. A detailed history may be obtained in 40 minutes from a reasonably communicative patient. With a difficult patient it may take much longer and more than one interview may be required, in which case the initial interview will concentrate on the presenting complaint and its history.

The Presenting Complaint

This is a statement, usually recorded in the patient's own words, of what he sees as his main complaint or problem.

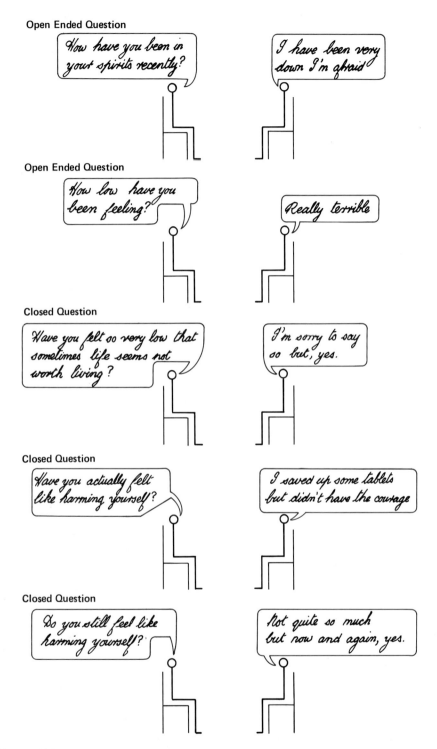

Fig. 2.3 *Establishing suicidal intent.*

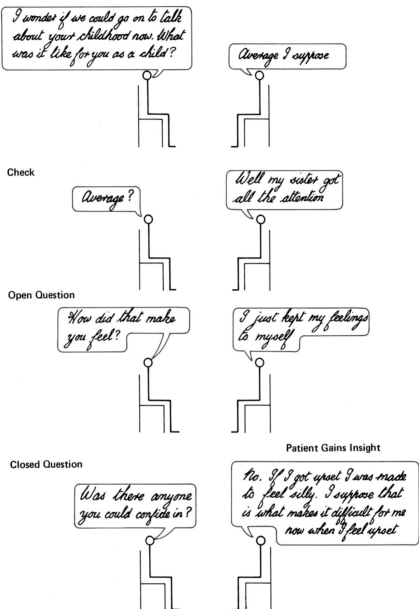

Fig. 2.4 *Open and closed questions related to childhood.*

The history of the presenting complaint

An elaboration of the presenting complaint with information on its severity and duration. Any events that may have had some influence on the development and continuation of the problem. How the complaint has affected the patient's relationships, work, interests, mood, appetite, sexual interest and sleep. Any other symptoms or complaints that he has been experiencing. Where a diagnosis of dementia is suspected, it is important to enquire into the patient's ability to wash, dress, find his way around, cook and manage his finances. The help of a reliable informant may be needed here. When a diagnosis of schizophrenia is suspected, it may be appropriate to ask about delusions and hallucinations. If the patient is depressed, the presence or absence of suicidal feelings must be ascertained.

Family History

The patient's family is taken in the order: mother, father, siblings. Their age, or age at death, the patient's age at their death, and cause of death. If alive, the proximity of residence and amount of contact with the patient. Their personalities and occupations. Any family history of psychiatric disorder. The question 'Has anyone in your family had any trouble with their nerves?' is useful here. Any other members of the family that the patient has been or is close to, for example, aunts, uncles or grandparents. The reaction of the patient to any bereavements experienced.

Personal History

Childhood

A chronological account of early childhood, schooling and adolescence, starting with birth. Relationships with parents and siblings. Relationship with peers. Academic achievement.

Occupation

Present occupation, job satisfaction and responsibility. Previous occupations with reasons for changing. If unemployed, reason for and adjustment to it. If retired, adjustment to it.

Sexual history

The patient may be reluctant to discuss this, particularly if the presenting complaint is not a sexual problem. Nevertheless, information on present and past sexual activity and satisfaction is important. For example, depression can cause loss of interest in sex, and sexual problems can cause depression and marital disharmony. An open ended question such as 'How has the sexual side of life been?' may allow the patient to volunteer any problems. Direct questions about masturbation, homosexuality and extramarital affairs may seem intrusive to the patient, who may deny problems and then feel guilty about having lied to the interviewer. This may close off areas that could be opened later when rapport has been more firmly established. If sexual problems are suspected but have not been volunteered, it may be better to ask an open ended question towards the end of the interview such as 'Is there anything else you would like to tell me that perhaps has been difficult or embarrassing for you to share?'.

Marital history

Account of present marriage or partnership. Previous marriages or close relationships with either sex. Occupation and personality of partner and harmony with him or her.

Children

Ages of children. Any behavioural or emotional problems. If the children are adult, how much contact the patient has with them.

Previous medical history

Accidents, illnesses and operations in chronological order. The impact any of these have had on the patient or his family.

Previous psychiatric history

Any psychiatric problems in the past, with details of duration, severity and treatment. Psychiatric notes and letters from the patient's general practitioner may need to be consulted.

Present medication

Record drugs and dosage.

Personality

This is an important part of the history and is an attempt to gain a picture of the sort of person the patient is when well. The mentally ill patient may have a distorted idea of how he is when well and to interview a reliable close friend or relative may be helpful. Aspects of personality may be considered under various headings such as personality traits, ability to get on with others, interests, habits, mood and religion. The patient or informant may be given a series of alternative words to describe the personality; for example, extrovert or shy, optimist or pessimist, perfectionist or careless, tense or relaxed, selfish or unselfish, self conscious or confident, open or secretive, worrier or easy going. It may also be helpful to ask for an account of a usual week in the life of the patient when well. Some elderly patients may have been depressed for many years and considerable perseverance on the part of the interviewer may be necessary to establish an accurate picture of the patient's previous personality. Careful enquiry into alcohol consumption should be included under personality. Finally, the patient should be asked if he has ever been in trouble with the law.

Social circumstances

An account of any financial problems. Type of housing and numbers sharing the accommodation.

At the end of the history the patient should be asked if there is anything more he wishes to mention that has not previously been covered.

THE MENTAL STATE EXAMINATION

This is a standardised recording of the patient's mental state as reported by the patient and as observed by the interviewer at the time of interview. Most of the mental state is recorded after the interview has ended, although the section dealing with disorders of thinking, and cognitive impairment may be recorded during the interview. The sections are as follows.

Appearance and Behaviour

The general attitude of the patient is commented upon; for example, whether he is friendly and cooperative, suspicious and hostile, tense or relaxed, inhibited or disinhibited. Is he dressed normally, cleanly, tidily? Does he seem restless and fidgety or does he sit abnormally still? Is he slow to respond and move (psychomotor retardation is a feature of depression) or overactive and distractible (a feature of hypomania)? Does he exhibit any involuntary movements such as tremor or dyskinesia, both of which may be due to side effects of antipsychotic drugs? Restlessness is of various types. It may be due to embarrassment, drug side effects or agitation. Agitation is a hand-wringing, perplexed type of restlessness accompanied by depressed mood.

Talk

The form of the talk is recorded, its speed, spontaneity, loudness, coherence, sudden change of topic, use of strange words and ability to keep to the point. Circumstantiality means undue description of trivial details and much delay in coming to the point. 'Perseveration' means that the same word or sentence is repeated often in response to a different question. 'Flight of ideas' occurs when the patient jumps from subject to subject, although the links between subjects are easily apparent. Where no links can be followed in the patient's talk, this may be due to 'formal schizophrenic thought disorder'.

Mood

This is a description of the patient's apparent mood. Does he look sad, sigh, burst into tears? Added to this is the patient's statement about his mood. Other mood states observed may be elation, fear, perplexity, anxiety. Incongruity of affect describes the mood of a patient whose expressed emotion does not seem to be appropriate to the topic of conversation, the extreme of which is laughing at sad events and crying about apparently happy events. 'Flatness' is used to describe lack of any emotion on the part of the patient. This may be a feature of schizophrenia.

Thought Content

The major pre-occupations, if any, of the patient are recorded here. Any abnormal thoughts are also recorded. Useful questions to allow the patient to describe abnormal thoughts are: 'Do you ever get the feeling that something strange is going on?' or 'Has anything unusual been bothering you recently?'. The abnormalities of thinking of particular interest are ideas of reference and delusions. Ideas of reference occur when the patient wonders whether other people are looking at him or talking about him. They become delusions of reference when he is convinced that this is so, that radio or television broadcasts have special meaning for him and so on. Delusions are abnormal beliefs, firmly held despite evidence that they cannot be true, which are out of keeping with the culture and education of the patient.

Disturbances of Perception

Patients may experience illusions, that is to say misinterpreted perceptions. More important are hallucinations, sensations experienced by the patient in the absence of any external stimulus. Most often auditory or visual, hallucinations can occur in any sensory modality. The patient may be asked about auditory hallucinations as follows: 'Do you ever hear noises or voices when there is no-one there?'.

Cognitive State

Cognitive function may be impaired in organic mental illness. The patient who can give a clear and accurate history is unlikely to have cognitive impairment. Where there is the slightest chance that the patient may have a poor memory or is unable to concentrate, formal testing must be undertaken. The patient with no cognitive impairment should be fully orientated in time, place and person. He should be able to repeat seven digits forwards and five backwards (digit span). A series of digits is given to the patient at one-second intervals, and he is asked to recall them. The unimpaired patient should be able to repeat accurately a name and address 5 minutes after being given the information, and should be able to give an accurate account of events in the preceding few hours. Problems with long-term memory are usually evident from the history. For elderly patients the Mental Status Questionnaire may be administered (Fig. 2.5). A score of less than seven is suggestive of cognitive impairment. It must be remembered that drugs can influence cognitive performance, and no test of cognitive function can discriminate between impairment due to depression and impairment due to organic illness.

What is the name of this town?
What is your address?
What year is it?
What month is it?
What is the date?
How old are you?
What month were you born in?
What year were you born in?
Who is the prime minister?
Who was the previous prime minister?

Fig. 2.5 *The Mental Status Questionnaire. Total score obtainable is 10; correct answer scores 1.*

Intelligence

This is the interviewer's subjective assessment of the patient's intelligence based on educational attainment and occupation, and is expressed as average, above average or below average. Remember that cognitive function varies directly with intelligence. A highly intelligent person will perform better on tests of cognitive function than a person of low intelligence.

Insight

The patient's ability to understand his symptoms in psychological terms. Some psychotic patients have little or no insight into the fact that they are ill.

THE FORMULATION

The formulation is a brief account of all the salient points in the history and present state of the patient. It may start with a comment on the personality of the patient and go on to outline predisposing and precipitating factors. It should contain a diagnosis (using the nomenclature of the International Classification of Diseases) and outline the features which support the diagnosis. A differential diagnosis should be mentioned and finally a plan for treatment and a statement of prognosis. A sample formulation is included (Fig. 2.6).

Personality	This is a 49-year-old woman of anxious personality. She had an unhappy upbringing, her mother dying when she was only eight
Predisposing factors	years old. Her father remarried but the patient had a poor relationship with her stepmother and felt that she was uncaring. She married at the age of 18, but her husband had several affairs and eventually left her when she was 30. Her father died about then and she became depressed, but improved with the help of antidepressants.
Precipitating factor	She remained well until four months ago when her only son left home to get married.
diagnosis	Since then she has developed a depressive psychosis with early morning wakening, loss of weight and appetite and suicidal feelings.
Differential diagnosis	The differential diagnosis includes depressive neurosis and underlying physical disease.
Treatment	She needs to be admitted to hospital in view of the suicide risk, and treated with antidepressant drugs. She also requires brief individual or group psychotherapy to help
Prognosis	her come to terms with her losses and enable her to adjust to being alone. She has coped well with previous stress and the eventual prognosis is good.

Fig. 2.6 *Sample formulation.*

ENDING THE INTERVIEW

If it is clear that history taking and assessment of mental state cannot be completed in a single session, the interview should be ended before time runs out and another appointment arranged.

When the interview has been completed, the patient is thanked for answering so many questions and asked if he has any questions of his own. He should be given a simple explanation of the significance of his complaints, together with a clear outline of what is proposed for the future – any further investigation, the type of treatment and so on. Reassurance, when justified, can also be given. The interview should end with a courteous farewell.

3

The Psychiatry of Physical Disease

Psychiatric symptoms in patients with physical disease may be produced in two ways. First, organic pathology may directly lead to impairment of cerebral function; such disturbances are called 'organic brain syndromes'. Second, the patient may fail to make a successful psychological adjustment to the stress of the illness, and react to it by developing psychiatric symptoms. These two mechanisms will be discussed in turn. It can be difficult to distinguish them from one another, and indeed it is not unusual for them to operate simultaneously in the same patient.

ORGANIC BRAIN SYNDROMES

Organic brain syndromes (organic psychoses) result from impairment of cerebral function by physical pathology. A wide range of pathological processes may be responsible. These include: structural damage to the brain (for example, the effects of head injury); metabolic disturbances arising from disease of other organs (for example, liver failure or hypoglycaemia); and poisoning by alcohol or drugs, including medically prescribed drugs. The clinical presentation depends on whether the underlying pathology is acute or chronic, and whether it affects the whole brain or a localised area. The symptoms are also influenced by the patient's cultural background and premorbid personality. An acute organic brain syndrome usually produces the clinical picture of 'delirium', a chronic one the clinical picture of 'dementia'. Occasional organic cases, however, present in a misleading fashion with symptoms suggesting a 'functional' psychiatric illness.

Delirium

Delirium (acute brain syndrome, toxic confusional state) is an acute syndrome in which impairment of consciousness is combined with abnormalities of perception and mood. The commonest cause in the UK today is withdrawal of alcohol from those who are physically addicted: delirium tremens. Other causes of delirium are listed in Table 3.1.

Clouding of consciousness is the essential feature. In mild cases the patient is muddled and unable to concentrate and becomes disorientated in time. Severely affected patients are obviously confused. The degree of impairment of consciousness fluctuates, so that the patient has some relatively lucid periods, but is more confused at other times, especially at night.

Thought and speech are incoherent, memory for recent events is impaired and perception is distorted so that people, objects and sounds are misidentified. In severe cases, transient delusions and hallucinations (especially visual) develop. In consequence the patient may be frightened, suspicious, restless and uncooperative.

The prognosis varies according to the

Table 3.1

Causes of Delirium

Cause	Examples
1. Infections	Encephalitis
	Meningitis
	Systemic infections
2. Vascular lesions	Cerebrovascular accidents
	Hypertensive encephalopathy
3. Metabolic	Hepatic failure
	Renal failure
	Electrolyte disturbance
	Porphyria
4. Endocrine	Thyrotoxic crisis
	Addisonian crisis
	Hyper- or hypoglycaemia
5. Toxic	Alcohol withdrawal
	Drug withdrawal
	Excess medication
6. Anoxic	Cardiac failure
	Respiratory failure
7. Epilepsy	—
8. Head injury	—
9. Vitamin deficiency	Thiamine (Wernicke's encephalopathy, beriberi)
	Nicotinic acid (pellagra)

underlying cause and whether this is amenable to treatment. Some patients recover fully. Others survive but have residual brain damage causing permanent dementia. Others become comatose and die.

Dementia

Dementia (chronic organic brain syndrome) is defined as an acquired global impairment of intellect, memory and personality, without impairment of consciousness. It usually develops gradually over a period of months or years, although a sudden deterioration caused by a change of environment or an intercurrent illness may first draw attention to the condition. Some cases follow an episode of delirium which leaves residual brain damage.

Memory impairment, affecting short-term rather than long-term memories, is usually the first symptom. It is accompanied by a general decline in intellectual ability. The patient gradually becomes forgetful, muddled, and less efficient than before. Thought becomes slow, repetitive, restricted in content and eventually incoherent, and corresponding changes are reflected in speech.

Changes in personality usually occur later, but are sometimes an early manifestation. Personality becomes coarsened or childlike, with lowered standards of cleanliness, social skills and consideration for others. Previous personality traits may become exaggerated. Behaviour consequently becomes disinhibited, sometimes to the extent that the patient commits a petty theft or sexual offence.

Mood changes are common. Depression, anxiety, irritability or perplexity may occur in the early stages in reaction to the patient's growing inability to cope with intellectual demands. Later, the brain damage results in emotional shallowness or lability, sustained depression, or inappropriate euphoria.

Delusions of paranoid type and hallucinations in the visual or auditory modality may develop in the later stages.

The changes are usually more obvious to other people than they are to the patient, who seldom complains about them spontaneously, but who may have enough insight in the early stages to attempt to conceal the disabilities.

Some causes of dementia are treatable, but most forms are progressive and irreversible. Senile dementia is the most common variety, and is followed in frequency by multi-infarct (arteriosclerotic) dementia (Chapter 7). The presenile dementias, which include Alzheimer's disease, Pick's disease, Jakob-Creutzfeld disease and Huntington's chorea, are far rarer. Alzheimer's disease is a familial condition which starts in middle age, and has a pathology identical to that of senile dementia. Pick's disease is also a familial condition starting in middle age and is characterised by cerebral atrophy most marked in the frontal and temporal lobes. Jakob-Creutzfeld disease does not run in families, but is believed to be caused by a virus. Affected patients develop rapidly advancing dementia and neurological abnormalities, at any age. Huntington's chorea is caused by an autosomal dominant gene. Symptoms usually include a combination of dementia and choreiform movements, and there may be other psychiatric abnormalities. The onset is usually in middle age when patients have already had children, of whom an average of 50% will carry the gene, but genetic counselling for members of affected families can reduce the incidence of the condition.

Dementia may be secondary to numerous other conditions, some of which are listed in Table 3.2.

The Amnestic Syndrome (see p.85)

Impairment of short-term memory, without significant impairment of other intellectual functions, may result from brain damage in certain sites. Damage to the hypothalamic–diencephalic region, including the mamillary bodies, most often results from thiamine deficiency in chronic alcoholism. Similar lesions may result from prolonged vomiting, malnutrition, or carcinoma of the stomach. Affected patients have a gross defect of recent memory so that all new information is forgotten within a few minutes, although immediate memory and long-term memory are both reasonably preserved. Some patients confabulate, that is, they attempt to compensate for the memory defect by elaborate falsification. This amnestic syndrome is also called Korsakoff's psychosis. Its development is sometimes preceded by an acute illness, Wernicke's encephalopathy, which has the features of delirium accompanied by nystagmus, ocular palsies, and often ataxia.

A similar short-term memory defect results from bilateral lesions of the medial temporal lobes,

Table 3.2

Causes of Dementia

Cause	Examples
1. Degenerative diseases	Senile dementia
	Presenile dementias
	Multiple sclerosis
	Parkinson's disease
2. Space-occupying lesions	Cerebral tumour
	Subdural haematoma
3. Infections	Neurosyphilis
4. Vascular lesions	Multi-infarct dementia
	Cerebrovascular accidents
	Systemic lupus erythematosus
5. Metabolic	Hepatic failure
	Renal failure
	Wilson's disease
6. Endocrine	Myxoedema
	Hypopituitarism
	Addison's disease
	Hyper- or hypoparathyroidism
7. Toxic	Alcohol abuse
	Drug abuse
	Excess medication
	Heavy metal poisoning
	Carbon monoxide poisoning
8. Head injury	—
9. Epilepsy	—
10. Vitamin deficiency	Thiamine
	Nicotinic acid
	B_{12}
	Folic acid

involving the hippocampus and hippocampal gyrus. Such lesions may result from encephalitis, cerebrovascular accidents, or neurosurgery performed to relieve epilepsy.

Focal Cerebral Pathology

Damage localised to a discrete part of the brain is often associated with a characteristic pattern of psychiatric symptoms and neurological signs.

Frontal lobe lesions

Personality changes are often the earliest

manifestation of a frontal lobe lesion. The patient's behaviour becomes disinhibited and childish, without consideration for the future consequences of his actions, or for the feelings of other people. Initiative and drive are reduced. Mood is often mildly euphoric. Incontinence is an early symptom and the patient is usually unconcerned about it.

Neurological manifestations occur later and include a grasp reflex, anosmia, optic atrophy, epileptic fits and eventually a contralateral spastic paralysis.

Temporal lobe lesions

Emotional lability, with a tendency to aggressive outbursts, is often associated with lesions of the temporal lobe. Symptoms of schizophrenia or affective psychosis less commonly occur. Bilateral damage to the medial temporal lobes, affecting the hippocampus and hippocampal gyrus, results in disturbance of short-term memory. Dysphasia and apraxia are associated with lesions of the dominant side, visuospatial disturbances with those of the non-dominant side.

Temporal lobe epilepsy often causes episodic psychiatric abnormalities, and the diagnosis is easily missed in cases without grand mal convulsions. The aura may include autonomic changes producing symptoms similar to those of acute anxiety: epigastric discomfort, tachycardia, breathlessness, dizziness, flushing or pallor. Perception is distorted, often causing feelings of depersonalisation and derealisation, of *déjà vu* or *jamais vu*. Visual, auditory, gustatory or olfactory hallucinations may occur. Thought may become incoherent, or focused upon inappropriate topics; memory is disturbed, sometimes with a re-experiencing of memories from the past. Intense affective experiences, usually unpleasant, may occur. The aura may be followed by a short period of organised yet inappropriate behaviour ('automatism'), or less often by a prolonged 'fugue' during which the patient wanders away from home,

unaware of his destination or even his own identity but apparently behaving normally. These phenomena may be called 'twilight states'. The patient is unable to remember them afterwards.

Associated neurological signs are a contralateral visual field defect, and mild contralateral paralysis or sensory loss.

Parietal lobe lesions

Parietal lobe lesions cause neurological rather than psychiatric disturbances. They include dysphasia, dyspraxia, visuospatial disturbances and body image disturbances. Examination shows cortical sensory loss. There may be a mild contralateral paralysis, and a contralateral homonymous hemianopia.

Occipital lobe lesions

Visual field defects, disturbed comprehension of visual stimuli, and visual hallucinations may result from damage to the occipital lobes.

Lesions of the diencephalon and brain stem

Lesions of the deep midline structures may cause a variety of psychiatric disturbances, depending on the exact site involved. Intellectual deterioration occurs early, there may be extreme lability of emotion, and personality changes of the same type as in frontal lobe lesions. Lesions of the mamillary bodies cause an amnestic syndrome. Hypersomnia, progressing to stupor and coma, may occur. Neurological signs include those of raised intracranial pressure, visual field defects if the optic chiasma is compressed, sensory disturbance if the thalamus is involved, and cranial nerve palsies accompanied by long tract signs if the lesion involves the brain stem. Lesions involving the hypothalamus or pituitary can cause endocrine changes.

Investigation of Organic Brain Syndromes

History-taking, mental state examination and physical examination are the first stages in the investigation of a patient thought to have an organic brain syndrome. The results of these determine which specialised tests need to be performed.

History-taking

Delirious patients are seldom capable of giving a full history themselves, so other informants need to be interviewed to elicit details of the present illness and of any recent medical symptoms, drug or alcohol abuse, or head injury which may be responsible for the condition. A psychiatric history is also required, because schizophrenia or manic episodes occasionally present as acute confusional states.

Demented patients who are not grossly confused may apparently be able to give adequate histories themselves, but often have impairment of memory, and poor insight into their altered behaviour and decreased intellectual abilities, which distort their own account. It is therefore essential to obtain a history from another informant, usually a close relative, as well. The medical history may reveal, for example, a family history of dementing illness, chronic alcoholism, past head injury, or symptoms of neurological, cerebrovascular, or endocrine disease. The psychiatric history may reveal symptoms of depressive illness, which often causes impairment of memory and concentration suggestive of dementia (depressive pseudodementia) in elderly patients.

Mental state examination (see p.16)

The delirious patient may appear physically ill, disoriented, and confused, and incapable of concentrating on the interview. Some patients show very little motor activity, others are restless and agitated. Talk is incoherent. Mood is often one of suspicion, hostility, anxiety or perplexity. Persecutory delusions may be present, but are usually vague and changeable. Hallucinations, most often visual, but sometimes auditory or tactile, may occur. Cognitive defects including disorientation, memory impairment and inability to concentrate are always present, but formal cognitive testing may be impossible.

The demented patient may not appear obviously ill or confused until the late stages of the disease. General appearance and behaviour may suggest organic pathology; for example, there may be evident weight loss, pallor, jaundice or premature ageing. Some physical conditions such as Parkinsonism or hypothyroidism produce a characteristic facial appearance, and neurological disease may cause obvious paralysis or abnormal movements. Grooming and hygiene are usually poor; incorrect arrangement of clothing suggests parietal lobe dysfunction. The patient may find it difficult to concentrate on the interview, become rapidly fatigued by questioning, or exhibit an inappropriate social manner. Talk may be off the point or frankly incoherent, and some patients keep repeating a single word or phrase (perseveration). Abnormalities of mood are frequent. Some patients show depression, anxiety or suspicion; others appear emotionally 'flattened' with minimal affective response; others have an inappropriate euphoria. Mood may fluctuate during the interview; for example, a mental challenge may precipitate a 'catastrophic reaction' of sudden anger or tearfulness. Vague ideas of being persecuted or robbed are common and may sometimes develop into fully formed delusions.

Formal cognitive testing is essential. Disorientation in time is an early symptom; disorientation in place and person may also be present. Attention and concentration, as assessed by the 'digit span' test or by simple arithmetic, may be impaired by incoherent thinking, easy distractibility or rapid exhaustion. Recent memory is often impaired in early cases. Long-term memory is well preserved until the late stages, although there may be amnesia for any episodes of delirium which have occurred in the past. General knowledge is tested by inquiring about current events, and questions on history or geography. The intelligence level, gauged by the interviewer's impression, is compared with the level which the patient's education and former employment would suggest.

Psychometric testing by a clinical psychologist is often a useful addition to the crude cognitive testing outlined above. Psychometric tests include those of intelligence, memory, abstract thought, and visuospatial ability. Such tests provide a numerical score for different cognitive abilities, and the results can be compared with those of the general population matched for age, or compared on different occasions in the same patient to chart progress. They can help to clarify the exact type of dysfunction present; for example, verbal ability, visuospatial ability or memory may each be selectively impaired. This information can be useful in locating the site of localised cerebral damage, and also identifies particular areas of severe handicap or intact skill which can be relevant to rehabilitation programmes. However, psychometric tests alone seldom provide a definite answer as to whether a case with mild cognitive impairment is 'organic' or 'functional'.

Physical examination

A full physical examination is routine for in-patients and should be performed on all out-patients in whom the history or mental state examination suggests organic cerebral dysfunction. Special emphasis should be placed on the nervous system, which is the most likely source of abnormality, but some organic brain syndromes result from non-neurological conditions.

Laboratory investigation

The type of laboratory investigation required depends on the history and examination findings.

In general, tests which are simple, cheap and involve little discomfort are commonly performed on all patients in whom there is a reason to suspect organic cerebral dysfunction, whereas more complicated, unpleasant or expensive investigations are reserved for patients in whom there is positive reason to suspect an abnormal result.

Any patient with delirium should have a full blood count and erythrocyte sedimentation rate (ESR), urea and electrolytes, liver function tests, blood sugar, blood alcohol level, chest x-ray, blood or urine screen for drugs, and urine tests for protein and micro-organisms. For patients with known or suspected dementia, this list should be extended to include thyroid function tests, serum B_{12} and folate, and serological tests for syphilis.

Many other more specialised tests may be indicated, and two frequently performed neurological ones, electroencephalography and brain scans, will be briefly described.

The electroencephalogram (EEG), a record of electrical activity in different parts of the brain obtained from electrodes placed on the scalp (Fig. 3.1), is abnormal in most patients with organic cerebral dysfunction, whatever its cause. It is especially useful as an aid to the diagnosis of epilepsy and of focal cerebral pathology. However, a normal EEG does not exclude organic cerebral pathology, and confusion can arise because patients with sociopathic personality disorder or 'functional' psychosis may show borderline EEG abnormalities. The EEG is altered by psychotropic drugs, and may be abnormal for several months following electroconvulsive treatment (ECT) (see p.128).

Brain scans include radioisotope scans and computerised axial tomography (CAT or CT) scans (Fig. 3.2). Radioisotope scans can detect a high proportion of cerebral tumours and other localised lesions. Computerised axial tomography scans are not available in all centres, but are preferable to radioisotope scans because they are non-invasive, and can reveal the presence of cerebral atrophy as well as localised lesions.

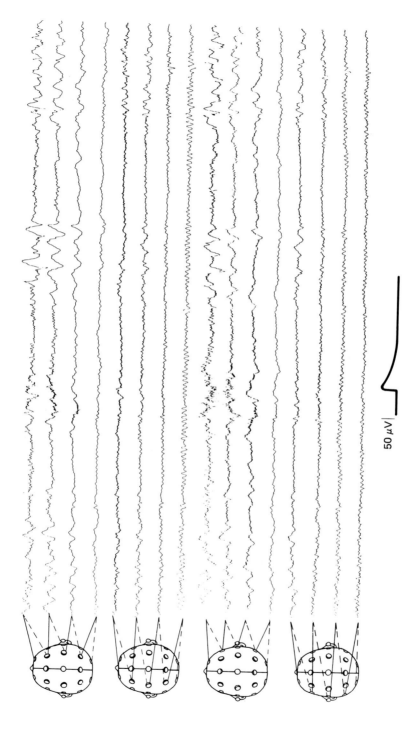

Fig. 3.1 Electroencephalograms (EEG). (a) High voltage spikes and slow wave complexes in right fronto-central region due to angioma. Normal activity on left.

50 µV

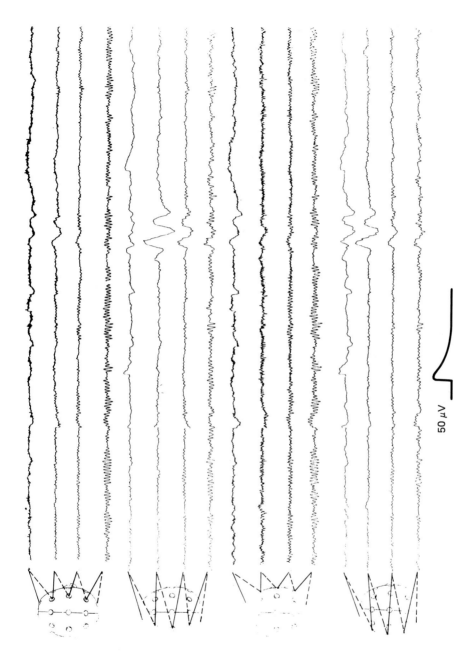

50 µV

Fig. 3.1 Continued. (b) *Left frontal abnormality due to a tumour.*

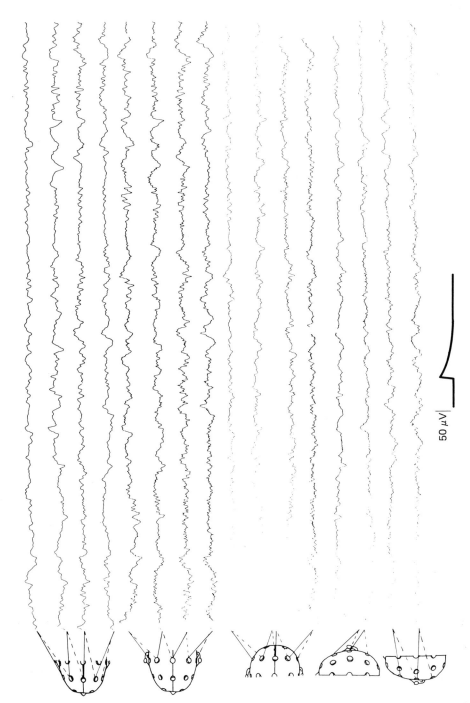

50 μV

Fig. 3.1 *Continued*. (c) *Slow waves, especially on right, due to a cerebral abscess.*

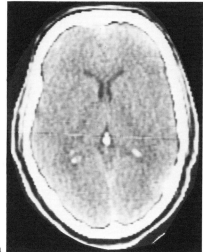

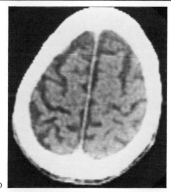

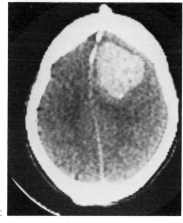

Fig. 3.2 *Computed axial tomograms (CAT scans) of the brain.* (a) *Normal cerebral cortex, at the level of the lateral ventricles. Note calcification of the pineal and of the choroid plexus.* (b) *Severe generalised atrophy of the cerebral cortex. The sulci over the convexities of both hemispheres are abnormally prominent.* (c) *Frontal meningioma, causing displacement of the falx.*

General Management of Organic Brain Syndromes

Whether or not the underlying pathology is amenable to treatment, optimal general management can often improve the condition of patients with organic brain syndromes.

Delirious patients may be less confused in quiet, well-lit rooms. They should be attended by a few familiar people, as encounters with a succession of strangers may add to their confusion or provoke paranoid reactions. Dehydration, electrolyte imbalance, infections and other physical complications require treatment. Patients who are restless, agitated or paranoid require sedation, and suitable drugs for this purpose include chlorpromazine, haloperidol and chlormethiazole. Anticonvulsants should be given if the patient has had fits. Care must be taken to avoid excessive medication, however, as this may increase confusion.

The management of the demented patient, who is usually elderly and physically frail, is discussed in Chapter 7 (p.71).

PSYCHOLOGICAL REACTIONS TO PHYSICAL ILLNESS

Some degree of emotional distress in reaction to serious physical disease is very common, but the majority of patients are not seriously incapacitated by such distress, and succeed in making a good psychological adaptation to their physical disabilities if these prove long lasting. There are other patients, however, whose emotional reactions are unusually intense, or apparently inappropriate in kind. Sometimes a full blown psychiatric illness is precipitated by the stress of a physical disease. Such 'maladaptive' responses usually cause patients added distress, and may interfere with their ability to co-operate with treatment. Some patterns of maladaptive psychological responses are described below.

Depression

Illnesses which entail some kind of loss for the patient are thought to be most likely to lead to depression. The most obvious examples are illnesses necessitating surgical removal of a valued part of the body; for example, amputation of a limb or mastectomy, but many other conditions also lead to loss in the form of impaired physical or social functioning. Mild unhappiness may be regarded as normal for a patient in such circumstances, but some patients develop formal depressive illness in reaction to them.

Anxiety

Anxiety is especially likely to be present in patients undergoing investigations to exclude a serious condition, those awaiting surgical operations or medical treatment of an unpleasant kind, or those suffering from conditions such as cancer or heart disease which involve a continued threat of recurrent illness or death. Like depression, anxiety of limited degree is a normal response to such circumstances, but in some patients it reaches extreme intensity and they develop symptoms of an anxiety neurosis. This may prevent them from co-operating with treatment.

Anger

Some patients unconsciously blame other people for their illness, and this is often manifest as hostility towards, and unjustified criticism of, medical and nursing staff.

Guilt

Patients may blame themselves for the development of the illness; for example, perceiving it as a punishment for some past misdeed. Guilt is often mixed with depression and accompanied by feelings of being a burden to relatives or a nuisance to staff, leading patients to minimise the severity of their symptoms or conceal them altogether.

Denial

Patients who employ the mental mechanism of denial unconsciously refuse to acknowledge the severity of their illness, either to themselves or to others. In mild degree this may have the beneficial effect of protecting the patient from distress, but it may also reduce compliance with treatment.

Welcoming of the Sick Role

To some patients, physical illness is not so much a source of distress as a source of unexpected benefits, such as increased attention from relatives, or escape from unwanted responsibility. Such patients' symptoms may be more severe or longlasting than their physical state can explain. This exaggeration of symptoms usually appears to result from unconscious mechanisms rather than from deliberate feigning of illness, and is sometimes termed 'hysterical'.

Management of Maladaptive Responses

These reactions can sometimes be prevented or modified if medical staff adopt a sympathetic approach to patients and their relatives, giving them as much information about the illness and its treatment as they seem ready to accept, and an opportunity to express their emotions and concerns. If symptoms of psychiatric illness develop, there is often a good response to the appropriate psychotropic drug.

EPILEPSY AND HEAD INJURY: TWO ILLUSTRATIVE EXAMPLES

Two common neurological conditions, epilepsy and head injury, have been selected to illustrate the mechanisms discussed above. Space does not permit description of the many other physical conditions which may be associated with psychiatric symptoms, but the more common ones are listed in Tables 3.1 and 3.2.

Epilepsy

Epilepsy affects about 6 per 1000 of the population. It was defined by the neurologist Brain as 'a paroxysmal and transitory disturbance of the function of the brain which develops suddenly, ceases spontaneously, and exhibits a conspicuous tendency to recurrence'. Attacks are usually associated with electrophysiological changes producing an abnormal EEG. Epilepsy may be generalised (grand mal or petit mal) or focal (e.g. motor epilepsy, temporal lobe epilepsy). In the majority of cases the cause is obscure, but about one-third are secondary to identifiable brain pathology.

Psychiatric disturbance is present in about 30% of all epileptics, and in at least 50% of patients with temporal lobe epilepsy or epilepsy secondary to a structural lesion. The disturbance may be a transient one occurring before, during or after the fit itself (peri-ictal), or present continuously (inter-ictal), and it may take the form of cognitive impairment, personality disorder, neurosis or psychosis. Organic, psychological and social factors all contribute to these disturbances.

Cognitive impairment

Most epileptics do not have cognitive impairment. Those without other evidence of brain damage have a distribution of intelligence within the normal population range. Some, however, show intellectual impairment from childhood, and a few develop dementia in adult life. The underlying brain damage, in cases of secondary epilepsy, is the most important cause. Other contributory factors in patients whose epilepsy is not well controlled are persistent electrophysiological disturbances present between fits, and cerebral anoxia during the fits themselves causing further damage to the brain. Anticonvulsant drugs, while helping to prevent the cognitive impairments which result from poor control of the epilepsy, may lead to such impairments themselves if given in excessive dosage. Lastly, children with epilepsy may have limited educational opportunities and so fail to fulfil their intellectual potential.

Personality disorder

There is an old-fashioned concept, derived from observations of institutionalised patients, of a typical 'epileptic personality' characterised by untrustworthiness, subservience, irritability, periodic aggression, and religiosity. It is now believed that personality disturbances occur in a minority of epileptics only, although they can be very severe. Personality disturbance appears to be most common in patients with secondary epilepsy, especially temporal lobe epilepsy. The brain damage responsible for the epilepsy is presumably the most important contributing factor in such cases, and is often associated with traits of irritability and emotional lability, and also with low intelligence which makes it more difficult for patients to adapt to their disabilities. Abnormal electrophysiological activity present between fits may make a further contribution. The surgical removal of a temporal lobe focus is often followed by improvement, especially a lessening of aggressive outbursts.

Psychological and social factors are also important in the aetiology of personality disturbance. Epilepsy still carries some stigma and from childhood onwards patients are treated differently from others. They are also debarred from many activities such as playing certain sports, driving, and have a limited choice of career. These restrictions may produce habitual feelings of isolation, resentment, or dependency.

Personality disturbance is sometimes exacerbated by anticonvulsant medication. For example, phenobarbitone can increase irritability.

Neurosis

Depression, anxiety, phobias, hysterical reactions and obsessive–compulsive symptoms are probably more common in epileptic patients than in the general population because of the greater degree of psychosocial stress to which epileptics are exposed. In some patients, mood disturbance and irritability is present for several days prior to a fit, and resolves afterwards.

Psychoses

Chronic schizophrenia and similar psychoses occur more frequently than would be expected by chance in patients with epilepsy, especially temporal lobe epilepsy arising from the dominant hemisphere. Paranoid schizophrenia is the commonest type and is characterised by the usual symptoms of delusions, hallucinations, passivity feelings, and thought interference. It usually develops some years after the onset of the epilepsy, and is often associated with some degree of cognitive impairment. More transient schizophrenia-like episodes lasting a few days or weeks and then resolving spontaneously may occur in patients with temporal lobe epilepsy, sometimes during a period when fits are not occurring and the EEG appears unusually normal. The mental experiences associated with the aura of temporal lobe epilepsy may also be reminiscent of those which occur in schizophrenia. Affective psychoses also occur more often than would be expected by chance in patients with temporal lobe epilepsy. Depressive episodes are more common than manic ones.

Suicide

Epileptics, especially temporal lobe epileptics, have a suicide rate about five times higher than the general population.

Head Injury

At least 1000 people each year in the UK are left severely disabled by physical handicaps, psychiatric disturbances, or both, as a result of head injury. Many others are affected to a lesser degree. Road traffic accidents are the commonest cause.

Most closed head injuries of any severity are followed by complete loss of consciousness, and then by a period of delirium with confusion, disorientation and cognitive impairment sometimes accompanied by acute psychiatric disturbance ('acute post-traumatic psychosis'). This may be exacerbated by complications of the injury such as haemorrhage or infection. The patient is usually left with amnesia for the accident itself, a short period beforehand, and a longer period afterwards. The duration of the unconsciousness, of the subsequent confusion, of retrograde amnesia and of post-traumatic amnesia all correlate with the severity of residual brain damage.

The patient's emotional reaction to the injury will be influenced by previous personality and by the circumstances of the accident; for example, whether any litigation or compensation payment is involved.

The occurrence of permanent brain damage and the development of maladaptive psychological reactions can both play a part in production of psychiatric disability. Such disabilities include cognitive impairment, personality change, psychosis, neurotic symptoms including the 'post-traumatic syndrome', or mixtures of these.

Cognitive impairment

Permanent intellectual deficit after a closed head injury is likely to occur if the post-traumatic amnesia exceeds 24 hours, especially in older patients. It usually takes the form of a global dementia involving all intellectual functions, and is often accompanied by neurological disabilities. Penetrating injuries, which are less common than closed ones, may produce selective cognitive impairments depending on the site of the damage: memory defects with damage to the medial temporal lobes, language difficulties with dominant hemisphere damage, visuospatial difficulties with non-dominant hemisphere damage. All but the most severe defects usually improve over a period of months or years.

Assessment requires thorough psychometric testing to identify both specific intellectual handicaps, and those functions which remain well preserved. Psychiatric assessment is also required, since depression or neurotic disability are often accompanied by apparent intellectual defects including forgetfulness and poor concentration. An individual rehabilitation programme can then be designed to re-educate the patient, making maximum use of his remaining physical and mental capabilities. Severely disabled patients may be best managed in a rehabilitation unit, where a multidisciplinary team including neurologist, physical medicine specialist, psychiatrist, social worker, physiotherapist, occupational therapist and speech therapist is available.

Personality change

Personality changes after head injury may be caused by organic brain damage, in which case they are often accompanied by cognitive impairments. Previous personality traits may become exaggerated or there may be a general coarsening of behaviour. Localised brain damage may cause characteristic changes; for example, frontal lobe damage causes apathy, disinhibition and euphoria, and damage to the amygdala produces a tendency to aggressive outbursts. The psychological reaction to the injury may account for other cases of personality change; for example,

patients may become chronically paranoid, depressed or irritable in response to the event and its adverse consequences. Such changes can sometimes be modified by counselling patients and their relatives or by the use of tranquillisers or antidepressants.

Psychoses

Schizophrenia, paranoid psychoses, and affective psychoses, usually depressive rather than manic, all develop slightly more often than would be expected by chance in patients who have had head injuries. Schizophrenia is associated with injury to the temporal lobes. Affected patients, however, are usually predisposed to psychosis anyway, as shown by a positive family history, previous personality abnormalities or previous psychotic episodes, so that the importance of the head injury itself is uncertain.

Psychoses are treated with the usual drugs and if these are not effective, ECT can safely be given to most previously head-injured patients.

Neuroses and the post-traumatic syndrome

Neurotic symptoms such as depression, anxiety, irritability, fatigue and insomnia are the commonest type of psychiatric disability following head injury. Hysterical or obsessive–compulsive symptoms are less frequent. Affected patients have usually had neurotic traits prior to the injury, and the symptoms are thought to result from the psychological reaction to the injury, since organic brain damage can seldom be demonstrated and since neurotic symptoms occur more commonly after mild injuries than severe ones.

Headache and dizziness, sometimes accompanied by forgetfulness, poor concentration and various neurotic symptoms, in patients who have had a head injury but in whom no organic brain damage can be demonstrated, is called the 'post-traumatic' or 'postconcussional' syndrome. This syndrome is assumed to have a psychogenic basis since it is more frequent after mild injuries than severe ones, and is more frequent if compensation for the injury is pending.

Neurotic symptoms may be helped by supportive psychotherapy aimed at providing insight and reassurance to both patients and relatives. Sometimes a period of observation in hospital helps to gauge the true extent of the symptoms if a difficult home environment is thought to be contributing to the disability, or if subtle organic impairments require investigation. Antidepressants or tranquillisers may relieve the symptoms. It is usually desirable for the patient to return to work at an early date, and for any litigation to be dealt with as soon as possible.

Suicide

Head-injured patients have a high suicide rate, and suicide is usually preceded by evidence of depression, personality changes or social problems.

4

Schizophrenia

Schizophrenia is a functional psychosis of uncertain aetiology which is often a chronic disorder and, in spite of advances in treatment, still sometimes disabling. There is no laboratory test for schizophrenia; it can only be recognised by its symptoms. These can conveniently be classified as positive (characteristic of acute episodes) and negative (defects of function characteristic of the chronic state).

EPIDEMIOLOGY

In the general population the life-time morbid risk (the risk of developing the illness at any time during a normal life span) for schizophrenia is just under 1%. The one-year prevalence of treated schizophrenia (the proportion of the population in contact with the psychiatric services with a diagnosis of schizophrenia at any time during a year) is between 0·2 and 0·4%, while the annual inception rate (the rate at which new cases occur during a year) is about 0·015%. The prevalence of schizophrenia is greatest in the lowest socio-economic class of the population, because the effects of the illness lead to a drift down the social scale for many patients.

The illness can begin at any age, but is rare before puberty. The peak age of onset is 20 to 40. Men tend to develop the illness at an earlier age than women, but the overall sex incidence is about equal.

CLINICAL FEATURES

Positive Symptoms

The most characteristic are a group of abnormal experiences described by Schneider as 'first-rank' symptoms because of their diagnostic importance. One or more of them occur in about 80% of cases. They include disturbances of the control of thought, delusions of control, primary delusions and certain types of auditory hallucinations.

The patient's subjective experience of his control of his thinking may be disturbed in one of three ways. He may experience thought insertion, when he is convinced that alien thoughts are put into his mind; thought withdrawal, when he believes that some outside agency is taking thoughts away from his mind; thought broadcasting, when his thoughts radiate from his mind and are received by other people.

Delusions of control refer to the patient's belief that his feelings, sensations, actions or bodily functions are influenced or controlled by an external force. This experience of no longer being a free agent is known as passivity.

A primary delusion occurs when a false belief erupts suddenly into consciousness with full conviction. In its most characteristic form it follows some neutral perception (delusional perception). One patient saw the postman open the garden gate and knew at once that a plot had been devised to poison him.

The characteristic types of auditory hallucination are three in number: loud thoughts (the patient hears his own thoughts spoken aloud); hearing one or several voices referring to the patient in the third person ('he' or 'she' rather than 'you', usually in a derogatory way); hearing voices commenting on the patient's behaviour ('He's getting out of his chair, going to the table, he's opening the drawer.').

All of these bewildering and alarming experiences may lead to the elaboration of secondary explanatory delusions. Thoughts are placed in the patient's mind by a laser beam; his actions are controlled by the CID computer; the voices are those of a gang of criminals who are spying on him and have bugged his house.

Schizophrenic patients may have many other positive symptoms. Most of them hear voices addressing them directly, commanding or deriding or even commending. Some patients describe somatic hallucinations, strange bodily feelings that are often attributed to external influence. Almost all patients have delusions that cannot be attributed to a disturbance of mood. These include delusions of persecution (he is being pursued by the secret service; someone is trying to kill him), of reference (there are special messages about him on the television, the headlines in the newspaper are about him), of grandeur (he is the emperor of the world). These delusions are often described in fantastic terms. Behaviour resulting from delusional beliefs or at the behest of voices may be violent or bizarre.

Catatonic symptoms, disturbances of motor function, are now much less common. The most characteristic is the maintenance for long periods of abnormal postures, whether self-induced or induced by the examining doctor. A patient might stand motionless or lie with his head a few inches above the bed for hours. Or he might keep his arm, say, in any position that the doctor puts it in, however unusual. Catatonic symptoms may occur as a result of brain disease and, in isolation, are not diagnostic of schizophrenia.

Depression of mood is common in acute episodes and may persist when more typical schizophrenic symptoms have subsided. Some patients are elated. More typical is emotional incongruity – the patient weeps unexpectedly or, more often, smiles or giggles inappropriately as if at a private joke. Emotional incongruity is characteristic of schizophrenia, but apparent incongruity may be due to anxiety or embarrassment in an interview.

Disturbance of thinking (thought disorder) occurs in some acute episodes. Logical associations between the patient's ideas are loosened and, as a result, his thought and speech become increasingly incoherent. Metaphoric and literal meanings become confused, words are used wrongly, sometimes new words (neologisms) are coined. One patient said, on a foggy day: 'Those fish swimming in that pea soup have been inserted and expopulated by all manner of devices to indicate the truth of the development of management and revolutionary theology'. The speech of a patient with severe thought disorder can be quite incomprehensible.

Negative Symptoms

These defects of function, characteristic of the chronic state, tend to persist but can be improved by rehabilitation (see below). Impairment of emotion and of drive are most important.

Emotional responsiveness is decreased; it may disappear entirely, so that the patient's facial expression is wooden and he uses none of the non-verbal means of communication that are so important in everyday social interaction. This symptom is called 'blunting' or 'flattening' of affect.

Drive, initiative and efficiency decrease. Many patients become capable only of increasingly menial jobs, eventually of no job at all. Severely affected chronic schizophrenics, if left to themselves, may do literally nothing all day. These symptoms are often accompanied by social withdrawal, an avoidance of social contact with other people.

These negative symptoms, a cause of grave disability when they are severe, are often accompanied by persistent thought disorder.

Cognitive Function

Schizophrenic symptoms occur in clear consciousness and, provided that the patient will co-operate, memory and orientation are usually found to be intact. In a minority of chronic patients, however, persistent defects of memory and of orientation are found. Such patients underestimate their ages and maintain that the date is several years earlier than it really is.

Types of Schizophrenia

Four sub-groups of schizophrenia have been described, although even the original workers realised that an individual patient might be classified in different sub-groups at different times in his illness.

Simple schizophrenia

This is the slow development of negative symptoms leading to persistent defects of function and social withdrawal without notable positive symptoms at any stage.

Hebephrenic schizophrenia

This is a combination of positive symptoms, emotional blunting and/or incongruity, and thought disorder with the eventual development of persistent negative symptoms.

Catatonic schizophrenia

Positive symptoms are combined with prominent catatonic symptoms including alternating excitement and stupor.

Paranoid schizophrenia

This is characterised by persistent delusions and, in most cases, auditory hallucinations with little or no thought disorder and few, if any, negative symptoms.

Late Paraphrenia

This term is applied to schizophrenic and paranoid psychoses which begin in old age (see p.68).

COURSE AND PROGNOSIS

The course of schizophrenia is very much influenced by the patient's psychosocial environment. In an unstimulating environment any negative symptoms will get worse. This used to be true of patients in chronic wards in mental hospitals, but it is also true of patients who spend most of their time alone in a bed-sitter or in a bedroom at home. Social stimulation improves negative symptoms, but too much stimulation and emotional interaction may precipitate or exacerbate positive symptoms. Some patients are intuitively aware of the dangers of over-stimulation and protect themselves by social withdrawal.

Some patients suffer from acute episodes only: perhaps only one episode, perhaps several episodes with reasonable mental health and no negative symptoms between episodes. A small proportion of patients develop florid positive symptoms which persist, in spite of treatment, for many years. At the opposite extreme other patients insidiously develop negative symptoms with scarcely any positive symptoms. Most characteristic is an initial episode of florid, positive symptoms followed by persistent negative symptoms, with further acute florid episodes, each marked by at least a temporary exacerbation of negative symptoms (Fig. 4.1).

The prognosis of schizophrenia has improved in recent years. Wing has summarised recent studies as follows: about one-quarter of schizophrenics will recover completely, another two-thirds will have relapses and may develop mild to moderate negative symptoms, while one-tenth will become totally disabled.

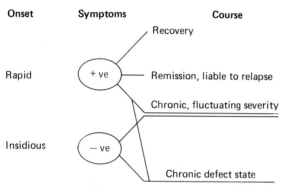

Fig. 4.1 *Simplified schema of course of schizophrenia. (Reproduced with permission from: Fairburn C.G. (1981). Schizophrenia. Hospital Update, 7: 1115–27.)*

MANAGEMENT

Medication

The first line of management is treatment with a neuroleptic drug; either an oral drug like chlorpromazine or trifluoperazine or, when compliance is doubtful, an intramuscular depot preparation such as fluphenazine or flupenthixol decanoate (see Chapter 13 for details). Neuroleptic drugs immediately control restlessness and excitement and, after several days, begin to suppress positive symptoms. Complete control of positive symptoms may take 6–12 weeks and sometimes only partial control is achieved. If the drug is withdrawn too soon, positive symptoms are likely to reappear. Patients whose symptoms are incomple-

tely controlled may need to continue medication indefinitely.

Neuroleptic drugs also protect against relapse if treatment is continued after an acute episode has subsided. However, because of the possibility of long-term unwanted effects, one does not want to give medication any longer than necessary. In the case of a patient who recovers completely with drug treatment, it is reasonable to withdraw the drug cautiously after a few months, especially if the clinical features suggested a good prognosis: such features include an acute onset, previous good personality and work record, the presence of affective symptoms (depression or elation of mood), life stress at the time of the onset. Relapse within two to three months after drug withdrawal suggests the need for prolonged prophylactic treatment. Relapse after several years of freedom from symptoms should be treated like a first episode: provided that symptoms disappear fairly promptly with medication, the drug can be withdrawn again after three to six months.

Rehabilitation

Neuroleptic drugs have little or no effect against negative symptoms. (One must remember that the sedative and extrapyramidal effects of a neuroleptic may mimic negative symptoms.) Patients with any serious degree of chronic defect and those with persistent or frequently recurring positive symptoms also need rehabilitation, preferably in a psychiatric rehabilitation unit. Here, in a structured environment, a programme can be tailor-made for the patient to enable him gradually to overcome or to compensate as many of his disabilities as possible, with the ultimate aim of leading as independent and rewarding a life as possible.

Techniques used in rehabilitation include counselling of both patient and relatives, training in occupation as well as in the skills of everyday living, and behavioural methods. Most patients also need continuing medication, usually in depot form. The treatment team includes the psychologist, occupational therapist and social worker as well as the doctor and the nurse. Rehabilitated patients need something to do and somewhere to live. Some patients can do a normal job, some can succeed in a sheltered workshop, others may attend a day centre where occupation is provided. Some patients return home (where the relatives as well as the patient need help and support). Others need a hostel or a group home (a house provided by a charitable housing association in which several ex-patients live), always with the hope of progression to greater independence in good lodgings or a flat. All too often the number of patients exceeds the amount of suitable accommodation available.

The essential sequel of rehabilitation is prolonged follow up, in which the psychiatric community nurse (who visits patients in their homes) has a vital role, to ensure that medication is continued where necessary, that support is always available and that relapse can be treated promptly (with urgent readmission when required).

Long Stay Patients

A small proportion of schizophrenic patients do not respond well enough to treatment and rehabilitation to achieve independence. They need medical and, especially, nursing care. This was traditionally provided in a long-stay ward in a psychiatric hospital, but it might be better provided in a hostel staffed by nurses in the community.

AETIOLOGY

Predisposing Factors

Schizophrenia runs in families, as Fig. 4.2 shows.

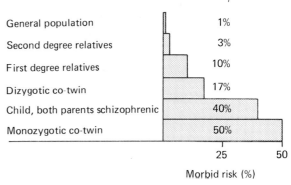

Fig. 4.2 *Morbid risk of schizophrenia in patient's relatives.*

The risk is greater in first than in second-degree relatives. It is greatest in the offspring of two schizophrenic parents and in the identical co-twin of a schizophrenic.

One viewpoint, which has given rise to several family interaction hypotheses, is that a person becomes schizophrenic because of pathogenic family, especially parental, influences during his formative years. Workers experienced in psychotherapy with schizophrenics and their families have described abnormalities in family structure, attitudes, expectations and modes of communication, claiming that these influences produce schizophrenia in a child. These hypotheses are at best unproven. The studies have usually been non-blind and uncontrolled and the abnormalities described have not been shown to be specific for schizophrenia.

Another view is that the liability to develop schizophrenia is inherited. This is supported by the difference in concordance rate for schizophrenia between monozygotic and dizygotic twins. (The concordance rate is the lifetime morbid risk of a disease in twins whose co-twins suffer from the disease.) The monozygotic twin concordance rate of only 50% (Fig. 4.2) shows that non-hereditary factors, of uncertain nature, determine whether schizophrenia ever becomes manifest. 'Cross-fostering' studies have shown that the offspring of schizophrenic parents retain their increased liability to develop schizophrenia even when adopted and reared by a normal family. The offspring of normal parents, adopted and reared by a family with a schizophrenic member, show no increased risk of schizophrenia. A study in Denmark compared a group of adoptees who had developed schizophrenia with a matched group of non-schizophrenic adoptees. An excess of schizophrenia and related disorders was found only in the biological (but not the adoptive) relatives of the schizophrenics.

The evidence is in favour of the genetic rather than the family interaction hypothesis, although the two are not incompatible. The mode of transmission is uncertain, but probably polygenic. People with a high degree of inherited predisposition are likely to develop schizophrenia in any environment, those with a lesser degree only as a result of exposure to other pathogenic forces.

Precipitating Factors

Patients with acute episodes of schizophrenia are much more likely than control subjects to have experienced a life event that required some adjustment to cope with it in the three weeks before the onset. It might be an unpleasant event, such as being made redundant, or a pleasant event, such as becoming engaged to be married. Recovered patients are more likely to relapse if they return home to live with relatives who express a lot of hostility, criticism or overconcern about the patient. Neuroleptic medication protects against both of these factors. Preliminary work suggests that relatives can learn to reduce their emotional expression and thereby to reduce the rate of relapse.

Biological Factors

Innumerable biological theories of schizophrenia have been constructed on what later proved to be inadequate grounds. The dopamine hypothesis is now in vogue; it postulates that positive symptoms of schizophrenia are due to overactivity of dopaminergic neurons or to increased sensitivity of dopamine receptors in the mesolimbic system. This neuronal system has its origin in cell bodies in the central midbrain and runs to limbic structures such as the amygdala, the nucleus accumbens and the limbic cortex (Fig. 4.3). The evidence for the hypothesis is mostly indirect. For example, antischizophrenic drugs block dopamine receptors; amphetamine causes central dopamine release and also causes a psychosis resembling acute schizophrenia. Amphetamine-like drugs may temporarily exacerbate positive symptoms in schizophrenics. Autopsy studies have found an increase in dopamine receptors, not entirely accounted for by medication, in schizophrenic brains. The dopamine hypothesis does not account for negative symptoms, which have been attributed to a deficiency in dopaminergic activity. Computerised axial tomography suggests that some chronic schizophrenics with severe negative symptoms have cerebral atrophy.

OTHER PARANOID PSYCHOSES

The concurrence of delusions and hallucinations that cannot be attributed to either mania or psychotic depression or to organic brain disease is usually attributed to schizophrenia. Some patients develop, often insidiously, delusions on a single theme without other schizophrenic symptoms and without any primary disturbance of mood. Examples include patients with persecutory delusions (paranoia), patients with the delusion that their spouses are unfaithful (morbid jealousy), patients who believe that they emit a smell, that their noses are too large, that they have some other physical abnormality (monosymptomatic hypochondriacal psychosis, which sometimes responds to pimozide, a neuroleptic). All of these types of delusion can occur in the setting of some

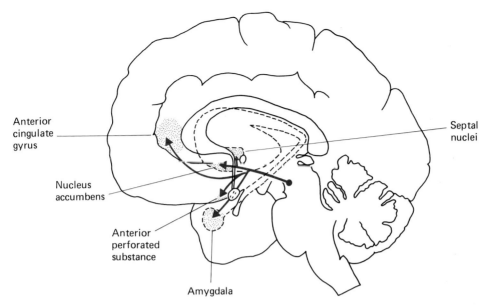

Fig. 4.3 *Diagram of the mesolimbic system.*

other psychiatric disorder. When they occur in pure culture they are usually classed as paranoid psychoses. Sometimes they occur transiently in the face of stress (this is especially true of persecutory delusions), but they are often chronic and unresponsive to treatment.

SCHIZOAFFECTIVE PSYCHOSES

This term is applied, with varying diagnostic criteria, to patients who show simultaneously clear features of schizophrenia and clear features of mania or psychotic depression. It is not clear whether they represent a separate group of disorders, a true blend of schizophrenia and affective disorder, or instances of misclassification. Prognosis is usually considered to be better than for schizophrenia but worse than for affective psychoses.

5

Affective Disorders

CLASSIFICATION

Affect is the psychiatric term used to describe mood. Although there are many abnormal types of mood, including fear, anger, anxiety, depression, suspicion and ecstasy, the term affective disorder is conventionally limited to the range of abnormal moods between mania at one extreme and major depression at the other. Mania is relatively uncommon outside psychiatric hospital practice but depressive illnesses are seen more frequently than almost any other psychiatric disorder. Unfortunately for the student, there is argument over the classification of affective disorders which leads to a confusing terminology. It is as well to be aware of the issues involved in classification at the outset so that confusion is avoided.

There are two views of affective disorder, which can be conveniently called broad and restricted. The broad concept regards any pathological disturbance of elevated or depressed mood as an affective disorder, whereas the restricted one only includes mania and major depression, which are collectively called the affective psychoses. The past history of illness is also relevant in classification. Affective psychoses in which mania and depression have both been present at different times are bipolar illnesses, and those in which only depression has been present are called unipolar ones. Patients who have had only episodes of

mania are usually regarded as having bipolar illnesses as manic episodes often appear earlier than depressive ones in the course of affective illness, but some have argued that unipolar mania is a clinical entity.

The student may also come across the adjectives 'endogenous' and 'reactive' to describe depression. These imply a link between aetiology and clinical features that does not exist. In this outdated terminology major depressive illness occurs without any precipitating cause and is therefore 'endogenous', whereas 'reactive' depression develops as a result of life stress, is of lesser severity and is equivalent to what is now called depressive neurosis or minor depressive illness. The reactive and endogenous labels will not be mentioned in this chapter again.

The important differences between the two classifications of affective disorder are shown in Table 5.1 and Fig. 5.1. We commonly refer to mood swings in describing the symptoms of affective disorder and it is therefore reasonable to measure these as if they were swings of a pendulum. If the swings are of only a few degrees, they are regarded as normal. If they are a little larger, they are regarded as cyclothymic personality disorder by the broad view but ignored by the restricted one. If they are larger still they become pathological and are classified as minor depressive

Table 5.1

Terminology of Affective Disorders

Nature of mood swing	Degree of swing	Broad view	Restricted view
Mania and depression	Large	Manic-depressive psychosis (Bipolar affective illness — manic and depressive phases)	Manic-depressive psychosis
Mania and depression	Small	Mild manic-depressive illness	Cyclothymic personality disorder
Mania only	Large	Manic-depressive psychosis	Manic-depressive psychosis (unipolar mania)
Mania only	Small	Not classified	Not classified
Depression only	Large	Major depressive illness	Unipolar depressive psychosis
Depression only	Small	Minor depressive illness	Depressive neurosis

illness by the broad view or depressive neurosis by the restricted one. (It is interesting that mild degrees of hypomania are not regarded as pathological and some would regard them as an ideal state of mind.) When the mood swings become very pronounced both the broad and restricted views coincide, and hypomania, mania and major depressive illness are unequivocal affective psychoses. Hypomania and mania are often used interchangeably but to be etymologically correct hypomania should be confined to less severe manic illness. One usage is to confine hypomania to episodes in which delusions (and hallucinations) do not occur.

The student may also come across the controversy whether there are one or two types of depression. This describes the difference between the broad view that all depression lies on a single continuum with typical cases of major and of minor depression at opposite ends (but with many intermediate cases showing mixed clinical features), and the restricted view, which holds that major depressive illness is one of the affective psychoses and is qualitatively different from minor

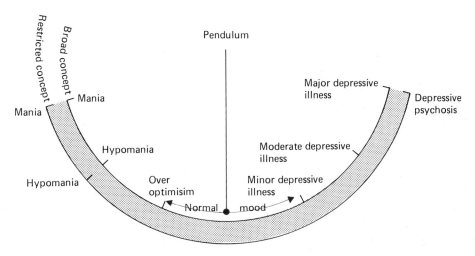

Fig. 5.1 *Broad and restricted concepts of affective disorder.*

depression, which is classified with the neuroses. Note that the difference between major and minor depressions is not simply one of degree; comparatively mild episodes of major depression occur, for example, in some bipolar patients, while minor (neurotic) depressions are occasionally quite severe.

To maintain consistency the terminology of the broad view will be used in the rest of this chapter. This means that minor depressive illness is discussed here instead of with the neuroses. It is important not to mix the terminology of one system with that of the other, and to realise that the merits of each system are finely balanced, so that either can be adopted.

EPIDEMIOLOGY

Mania and hypomania are much less common than pathological depression. Studies of referral to psychiatrists (which include almost all patients with mania) show that the annual prevalence is 3 per 10 000 (0·03%), whereas major depressive illness is more than ten times as common, with an annual prevalence of 2·5 per 1000 (0·25%). The rate for minor depressive illness is 3 per 100 (3%). In general population surveys, the figures for depressive illness become even greater; in one recent study 17% of women in an urban area experienced depressive symptoms in the course of a year. These figures, if replicated, would make depressive illness the most common psychiatric disorder. All forms of depression are at least twice as common in women than in men.

AETIOLOGY

Genetic Factors

Genetic studies consistently show that there is a stronger hereditary component in bipolar disorder than in unipolar depressive illness, and that the genetic predisposition to minor depressive illness is much less than that to major depressive illness. There is a higher concordance rate in monozygotic than in dizygotic twins for both unipolar and bipolar affective disorder, while the concordance rate in monozygotic twins is higher for bipolar than for unipolar affective disorder (Table 5.2).

Table 5.2

Genetic Factors in Bipolar and Unipolar Affective Illness

	Bipolar	Unipolar
Concordance in monozygotic twins (%)	70	48
Concordance in dizygotic twins (%)	20	14
Risk in first degree relatives (%)	15	10

Because the concordance rate for bipolar disorder in identical twins is less than 100%, it has been suggested that the illness is transmitted by a single dominant gene of incomplete penetrance. An alternative explanation is that liability to develop the illness is determined by several genes working together (polygenic inheritance). One study of adoptees (cf p.40) also suggests that inheritance is of major importance in the transmission of bipolar affective disorder.

Biological Factors

The biochemical aspects of affective disorder are difficult to interpret aetiologically because they can often be regarded as secondary features that follow the onset of the disorder rather than cause it. The most common biological hypothesis of affective disorder is the monoamine hypothesis, which states that depressive illness is caused by a relative deficiency of central monoamine neurotransmitters (mainly noradrenaline and 5-hydroxytryptamine) and that mania is caused by a relative excess of the same monoamine. The best evidence for the hypothesis is that severe depression can be caused by drugs that reduce cerebral monoamines. These include the hypotensive drugs reserpine and methyldopa, which reduce blood pressure by catecholamine depletion. The drugs used to treat depression generally increase the concentration of monoamines at receptor sites. Occasionally their use leads to attacks of mania. Electroconvulsive therapy (ECT), which may also precipitate manic episodes, is thought to act by altering receptor sensitivity to monoamines. Indeed, more recent monoamine theories suggest that deficiency of either noradrenaline or 5-hydroxytryptamine leads to increased sensitivity of other receptors in the brain, which in turn is responsible for many of the symptoms of depression. Mania is thought to be associated with increased dopaminergic activity as well.

There is increased cortisol production in about half the patients with major depressive illness. This appears to be a secondary feature of the disorder, but in medical conditions in which excess cortisol is produced such as Cushing's syndrome (or in high dose steroid therapy) a severe form of depressive illness may result. The synthetic steroid dexamethasone fails to suppress cortisol secretion in some depressed patients but not in others, and this is sometimes used as a diagnostic test for depressive illness. Other organic precipitants of depression include infectious mononucleosis, hypothyroidism and vitamin B_{12} deficiency.

Social Factors

The importance of social factors in the causation of depression has been underlined by the work of the sociologist, George Brown. Loss of a parent during childhood may lead to a higher risk of depressive illness in adult life, while other forms of loss are also precipitating factors. Studies of patients with both major and minor depressive illness have shown that they are much more likely than control subjects to have experienced one or more severely threatening life events during the months before the onset of the illness. The interval between life event and onset tends to be greater in major than in minor depression. Other depressions develop against a background of chronic severe difficulties; with money, with housing, with a spouse and so on. In women at least certain factors protect against depression; these include having a job and having a confiding relationship with a husband or boy friend.

In many cases the threatening life event can be regarded as an actual or threatened loss. Loss covers many factors, including lack of contact through separation (e.g. following divorce), being made redundant, or a drop in social status as well as the more obvious ones of bereavement, etc. Short-lived feelings of depression are common after loss, and are not in themselves abnormal. Indeed, the expression of normal grief is considered healthy and allows adjustment to the loss to take place. The incorporation of mourning as an acceptable ritual for expressing grief in the social fabric of most societies indicates the need for grieving after loss.

Grief can change into depression, particularly if it is not really expressed, and the dividing line between 'normal' grief and pathological depression is not easy to draw. Both include the symptoms of depression but there are some important differences; these are summarised in Table 5.3.

Social isolation is also an important aetiological factor in depression, particularly in relationship to suicide. Isolation is a common consequence of separation and loss, and the person who suffers a depressive illness is more likely to make a serious suicide attempt if alone and isolated than if he is part of a close social network. Depressive illness is also less common in communities that show marked social cohesion. Age is relevant in that older patients are much more likely to present

Table 5.3

Differences Between Grief and Depressive Illness

'Normal' grief	Depressive illness
Immediately follows an adverse life event	Delay between adverse life event and onset of symptoms
Rarely lasts more than a few weeks	Persistent for weeks, months or years
Adjustment to and acceptance of the loss occur during recovery	Denial of the loss and refusal to accept its implications are common features
Experience of grief open and uninhibited	Experience of grief limited and sometimes absent

with symptoms of major depressive illness than younger patients. The reason for this is not known.

Manic illness is not clearly related to environmental factors in the same way as depression, although clinical experience suggests major life events sometimes trigger episodes of illness.

CLINICAL FEATURES

Mania

The major clinical symptoms of hypomania and mania are elevation of mood, increased self-confidence and accelerated psychomotor activity. These are accompanied by unrealistic plans and impaired judgement and awareness of illness (insight) is often absent. When hypomania progresses to mania these features are more pronounced. Although the key symptom of mania is elevation of mood, it should be realised that this is not always a state of infectious euphoria. The manic patient is frequently prevented from carrying out his unrealistic plans by friends and relatives and so becomes irritable and angry when thwarted. Because he cannot understand the reasons for this he may also feel that he is being unfairly discriminated against and become critical

and paranoid. In some patients irritability is much more evident than euphoria. Other patients show brief episodes of depression, lasting usually a few minutes, and sometimes accompanied by tears and depressive thoughts ('microdepressions').

An increase in psychomotor activity is almost invariable in mania. It shows itself in a rapid progression of thoughts (pressure of thought). These spill over in a stream of talk that at first seems to be completely disjointed but on closer examination reveals links from the different themes. Thus, the speech fragment 'Don't tie me up doctor. Don't try me in Court, the Royal Court, give me the Queen's pardon' is a short example of the talk of mania, formally termed 'flight of ideas'. It demonstrates the rapid switching from one subject to another, but on closer examination there are detectable links in the content of the speech. Thus, the link between 'tie' and 'try' is in the sound of the word (clang association) and a pun on the word 'court' provides the connection between being charged for an offence and royalty. These links are not present in the fully developed thought disorder of schizophrenia. Manic patients are very distractable and find it difficult to stick to any one theme for more than a few seconds, and even the sound of the words is enough to start them off on a new track. This distractability also shows itself in heightened awareness of environmental stimuli and in great restlessness and alteration in behaviour with inability to settle to any one task.

In mania, energy is abundant and apparently inexhaustible. The patient needs little sleep and often causes major disruption by his noisy activities in the small hours. Sexual interest and activity is greatly increased and promiscuity can be a problem. Because the patient is disinhibited he may also drink excessively and spend money with reckless extravagance, perhaps spending his life savings in a few days.

In more severe cases, grandiose delusions are present. Often the patient claims to have special powers, a special identity, or a special mission and demands to be treated with appropriate respect. In seconds the mood can change from jocularity to anger if this respect is not forthcoming. Paranoid delusions may also be noted but these are obviously secondary to the mood disturbance. The delusions are sometimes accompanied by visual and auditory hallucinations such as the appearance of angels and voices telling the patient that he has been chosen for a special task. Eating and drinking become unimportant in mania and occasionally patients can lose a great deal of weight and become dehydrated. As insight is usually lacking in mania, compulsory admission to hospital is often necessary.

It is usually easy to diagnose mania but, if paranoid features are marked and if flight of ideas is extreme, schizophrenia may be wrongly diagnosed. If all the behavioural disorders, delusions and hallucinations are consistent with an elevated mood and excessive psychomotor activity (i.e. are affectively based), then the diagnosis of mania should be made.

Major Depressive Illness

In major depressive illness, or depressive psychosis, the clinical picture is the opposite of that seen in mania. The mood is continuously depressed, psychomotor activity slowed and self confidence is reduced to such an extent that the patient feels worthless and a burden on his family and society. A distinction is often made between retarded and agitated depressive illness; in both disorders there is similar depressed mood and associated features, but the slowing is more marked in retarded patients while agitated patients show purposeless motor overactivity such as pacing up and down, rocking to and fro, wringing hands and so on. Very rarely, the patient may show no overt evidence of depressive mood despite some psychomotor retardation and in the rare 'smiling depressive' the mood is superficially cheerful. Psychomotor retardation (the adjective

psychomotor is usually advisable so that intellectual retardation is not implied) is shown by limited spontaneous movements of the limbs, face and body (in this respect severe depressive illness is similar to Parkinson's disease), greatly reduced speech with no spontaneous conversation and monosyllabic replies to questions (poverty of speech) with a long latent period between question and answer. In very severe cases this progresses to depressive stupor when the patient sits with his eyes open but shows no other movement.

There is marked pathophysiological disturbance in fully developed major depressive illness. Appetite is not just reduced, it becomes nonexistent and patients complain that their food no longer has any taste. There is considerable weight loss as a result, often more than 10 kg. Sexual interest and activity is reduced or non-existent and in milder cases impotence is common. There is an unusual form of sleep disturbance that some regard as almost pathognomonic of depression, that of early morning waking. The patient gets off to sleep without any difficulty but wakes in the early hours of the morning feeling depressed and wretched, and is unable to get to sleep again (it is no coincidence that the early hours of the morning are the peak hours for successful suicide). Early morning waking is often accompanied by a diurnal mood swing, with depressed mood and retardation being at their most prominent in the early morning and then improving at least a little as the day goes on.

Cognitive testing in severe depressive illness often suggests organic impairment. Because the patient's attention, concentration and registration are poor he is unable to carry out simple mathematical and deductive tasks and is sometimes disorientated. This depressive 'pseudodementia' should not be confused with true dementia; when the abnormal mood is reversed, normal cognitive function returns.

Delusions are frequent and hallucinations occasional in major depressive illness. The patient's feelings of worthlessness and uselessness can become so pronounced that he blames himself for everything that has gone wrong, even matters that are completely beyond his control. When these become fixed beliefs they are described as delusions of guilt and indicate that treatment is needed urgently. Otherwise, there is a strong risk of successful suicide. Sometimes the patient's delusions may extend to others who are close to him. In an attempt to reduce the alleged suffering of the relative he or she is murdered and then the patient commits suicide. This is a particular risk in puerperal depressive illness. Delusions of poverty may also be present, when the sufferer believes himself to be bankrupt despite having healthy assets. Hypochondriacal delusions are also common; there is a frequent complaint that the stomach and gut is blocked up and fears of cancer are common. Sometimes the patient believes that parts of his body or things about him do not really exist and constitute a vacuum; these are called nihilistic delusions. Auditory hallucinations are also experienced, when the patient hears voices criticising him and often exhorting him to suicide. Insight is often lost in the most severe forms of depressive illness and compulsory admission to hospital may be necessary.

Minor Depressive Illness

This presents quite a different picture. Although depressed mood is prominent, it is not all pervasive, and the patient may be cheered up temporarily when placed in the right setting. Although energy is reduced and the patient often complains that everything is an effort, there is no psychomotor retardation and the patient can appear quite normal to an external observer. There is no early morning waking and the patient more commonly experiences initial insomnia, lying awake for one to two hours before falling asleep. He may awake subsequently in the night but go back to sleep again quickly. There is usually no diurnal mood swing, although sometimes a mood

pattern is shown that is opposite to that of severe depression. The patient wakes up feeling well but, as the day goes on, he is reminded of the events that cause him to feel depressed and he feels worse at the end of the day.

Appetite varies between anorexia and overeating. Many overweight patients first become obese after a loss that leads to mild depression, after which solace is sought in food. Delusions and hallucinations are not found in mild depressive illness. The patient may commit suicide but attempted suicide (parasuicide) is more common.

Mixed Affective Disorder

This is an unusual form of affective disorder in which both manic and depressive features are seen together. The patient rapidly alternates between a state of excitement and overactivity and severe depression with suicidal thoughts. Insight is almost completely lacking.

DIAGNOSIS OF AFFECTIVE DISORDER

The chief differences in clinical features between the two types of depression and mania are shown in Table 5.4. It will be noticed that the manic and depressive features are almost exact opposites of each other. Minor depressive illness presents a picture which is different from that of major depression.

The assessment of affective disorder is not difficult provided that it is done systematically. A suggested scheme to follow is shown in Fig. 5.2.

The mood disturbance is usually the most prominent feature and immediately arouses the suspicion of affective disorder. If this has occurred in a setting of acute loss, such as the death of a close relative, it will often be regarded as normal grief and not a true affective illness. If the duration of mood disturbance is longer and severity of

Table 5.4

Comparison of Clinical Features in Mania and Depressive Illness

Clinical features	Minor depressive illness	Major depressive illness	Mania and hypomania
Movement	Normal	Retarded or agitated	Accelerated
Speech	Normal	Reduced (poverty of speech)	Increased (pressure of talk, flight of ideas)
Energy	Reduced	Greatly reduced	Increased
Sleep disturbance	Variable	Normal onset of sleep Waking in early hours feeling low-spirited	Variable, but sleep less than normal without increased tiredness
Appetite and weight	Little change	Reduced	Variable
Libido	Little change	Reduced	Increased
Delusions	Absent	Occasional (guilt, poverty, hypochondriacal)	Common (grandiose)
Hallucinations	Absent	Occasional (usually auditory)	Occasional (auditory and visual)
Insight	Present	May be absent	Often absent

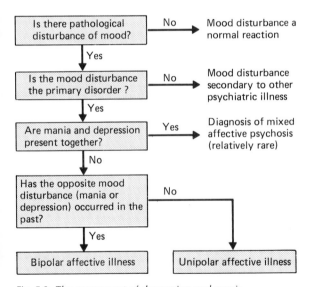

Fig. 5.2 *The assessment of depression and mania.*

symptoms more pronounced, the mood is regarded as pathological. It is a mistake to assume that pathological depression necessarily indicates a diagnosis of affective disorder. Secondary mood disturbance is frequent in schizophrenia, alcoholism and drug withdrawal syndromes, obsessional neurosis and organic (including drug-induced) psychoses. It is not an easy task to decide if the mood disorder is the primary event in the illness, but if all the features of illness are consistent with the mood disturbance an affective disorder is the likely diagnosis.

The most frequent differential diagnoses of mania are drug-induced psychoses (e.g. LSD, amphetamines) and acute schizophrenia, in which there is great pressure of talk and elated mood but the infectious warmth of true mania is lacking. Severe depressive illness can be confused with early dementia, particularly if 'pseudodementia' is present, and with obsessional neurosis, as obsessional symptoms are frequently present in severe depression, and improve as the depression lifts. In cases of doubt it is probably better to treat an obsessional patient with depressive symptoms as primarily depressed unless there are strong indications otherwise.

Once the rare diagnosis of mixed affective psychosis has been excluded, the bipolar/unipolar distinction is made. In some respects this decision is provisional only as it is always possible at a later stage in illness that the opposite mood pole may present. The subdivision of unipolar affective illness into major or minor forms is easy if the patient presents the classical features indicated in Table 5.4, but if there is an overlap of clinical features it is a different matter. As a working rule, if more than one of the features below 'Energy' are present, and are typical of a major depressive illness, then this should be the diagnosis — even if other minor depressive symptoms are present. The significance of making this distinction will be apparent when treatment is discussed.

TREATMENT OF AFFECTIVE DISORDERS

The milder forms of depressive illness are best treated by psychotherapeutic measures. These are particularly appropriate when the depressive disturbance follows loss. Once the disturbance has become too severe or prolonged to be regarded as normal grief (Table 5.3), adjustment to the loss can be regarded as maladaptive and treatment is needed. At its simplest level the psychotherapy involves a sensitive exploration of the circumstances of the loss with the patient. By reactivating the unpleasant memories in a supportive way they can be brought into full consciousness and their implications accepted without denial or guilt. This procedure is often termed 'working through' the depression. Additional aids to this process have been introduced from behaviour therapy. For example, in the procedure called 'guided mourning' the patient is asked to carry out tasks such as visiting the grave of a dead relative regularly or looking at photographs of the deceased and saying 'goodbye'. The same aim applies to all these treatments; to bring the feelings of grief out into the open so that the loss can be accepted and a positive readjustment made.

Removal from the source of the depressive disturbance, help with chronic difficulties and other measures based more on common sense than specialised knowledge may also be very effective treatment. These must not, however, be used only as a means of escape from the stress. Depression arising through pressures at work may be temporarily relieved by a holiday, but resolution of the problem can only be achieved by a change at the workplace. Frequently the environmental and social changes indicated can only be made after involving other people. Although the patient has to make the important decisions himself, the doctor can be of value in pinpointing the issues that are aggravating the depressive disturbance.

Drug treatment is indicated if social and psychotherapeutic measures have failed or are impossible to put into practice (e.g. getting a depressed and demoralised unemployed man back into work again). It is also appropriate if the depressive illness does not appear, after full enquiry, to have any obvious antecedents or precipitants. Often antidepressant drugs are given too readily because they are easier and less time consuming to administer than the other treatments. If the decision to prescribe drugs is made, the other forms of therapy should still be used when the time is right. Treatment in psychiatry used to resemble a battleground in which the warring armies of psychotherapy, behaviour therapy and 'organic' treatment were in constant conflict, but it is now realised that these theoretically distinct treatments combine with each other well.

Tricyclic antidepressants, the newer antidepressants such as mianserin, nomifensine, maprotiline and trazodone, some antipsychotic drugs such as flupenthixol, and monoamine oxidase inhibitors have all been used to treat minor depressive illness of lesser and greater severity. In general they are much less valuable than in major depressive illness. There is little difference in efficacy between the different antidepressant drugs in 'pure' forms of depression. When, as frequently happens, the depressive symptoms are mixed with generalised anxiety, agoraphobia and social fears, it is better to choose a monoamine oxidase inhibitor or a sedative antidepressant such as trimipramine or amitriptyline. It should be remembered that all the drugs take between 10 and 40 days to show their full clinical effects and the patient should be warned about this when the drugs are prescribed. The use of drugs is discussed in more detail in Chapter 13.

The choice of treatment is different in major depressive illness. Such patients are not amenable to psychotherapy or behaviour therapy and physical treatments are the ones of first choice. Electroconvulsive therapy (ECT) is the most rapidly acting antidepressant treatment and may be used first if (a) the patient is seriously suicidal and a delay in the onset of therapeutic effects is considered too great a risk, (b) the patient is refusing to take food or drink (and antidepressant drugs), or (c) the patient is in a depressive stupor. Such patients are invariably treated as inpatients and often require compulsory admission.

Under most circumstances treatment with one of the tricyclic antidepressants or newer antidepressant drugs is usually given first. The choice of drug will be governed primarily by the differences in unwanted effects (see Chapter 13) as there are no significant differences in efficacy or time of onset of therapeutic effects between these antidepressants.

Mania and hypomania are also not amenable to psychotherapy. Both the antipsychotic drugs and lithium carbonate are effective treatments, but the former are usually preferred because of fewer dangers of toxicity. If lithium carbonate is used to treat mania, higher serum levels are needed (above 1·0 mmol/l) than in the prophylaxis of manic-depressive psychosis and at these levels it is easy to stray into the range at which toxic effects become apparent (above 2·0 mmol/l) (see p.125). When antipsychotic drugs such as haloperidol and chlorpromazine are used first, they usually need to be given in high doses, and patients need to be observed closely for extrapyramidal side effects. If these become manifest an anti-Parkinsonian drug will be needed. Most attacks of mania are relatively short-lived and the first sign that an episode is coming to an end is that the patient becomes drowsy and lethargic on a dose of drug that formerly seemed to have no effect.

The choice of initial treatment for the different types of affective disorder is summarised in Table 5.5, which does not include preventive drug therapy. Prophylaxis of recurrent major depressive illness and mania is often necessary if attacks are more frequent than once every two to three years. Lithium carbonate is the drug of choice in bipolar affective psychosis and both tricyclic antidepressants and lithium carbonate appear to be equally effective in the prophylaxis of unipolar depressive illness. There is no reason why patients should not live normal lives free of untoward effects on long-term drug prophylaxis, but only a small minority of patients with affective disorder come into this category.

Table 5.5

Treatment of Affective Disorders

Treatment	Minor depressive illness (Depressive neurosis)	Major depressive illness (Depressive psychosis)	Mania and hypomania
First choice	Psychotherapy and behaviour therapy	Tricyclic or newer antidepressant drugs	Antipsychotic drugs
Second choice	Social and environmental manipulation	Electroconvulsive therapy	Lithium carbonate
Other effective treatments	Monoamine oxidase inhibitors Tricyclic antidepressants	—	—

6

Neurosis and Personality Disorder

Principal Characteristics

Together these two groups of psychiatric disorder constitute by far the largest portion of psychiatric disorders, accounting for approximately one-half of all admissions to psychiatric hospitals, three-quarters of all patients seen in outpatient clinics and over 90% of psychiatric disorders seen in general practice. Unfortunately, as with other psychiatric disorders, the terminology of neurosis and personality disorder is open to dispute. This will be apparent from the previous chapter in which so-called depressive neurosis as been discussed with the affective disorders.

Neuroses are mental disorders which have no organic basis (i.e. are 'functional'), which differ from more serious mental disorders (psychoses) in that insight is usually maintained and the main complaints are those of symptoms that are immediately understandable to someone with no mental disorder. In other words, these symptoms are quantitatively different from normal experience rather than qualitatively different. Thus, distorted perception and belief do not occur in neurotic disorders and the personality remains intact and well organised. In lay terms, neurotic patients are perceived as normal (or nervous) and psychotic patients as mad.

Personality disorders may be associated with neurotic symptomatology but the main handicap is that of maladaptive behaviour which produces impaired social and personal adjustment. Although each person has a unique personality, there are certain features, called traits, which are more prominent than others. Normally these traits are not expressed in situations where they are inappropriate but in personality disorder they dominate behaviour and cause suffering both to the patient, his family and, ultimately, society. Personality development occurs in the early years of life but can be modified in adolescence and early adult life. After this time the personality pattern becomes relatively ingrained and is difficult to alter, although some changes may occur with age. Personality disorders therefore tend to be long-term handicaps with a history of chronic social maladjustment.

The chief difficulty in differentiating neurotic from personality disorders is when the neurosis is a chronic one. Such neuroses frequently alter behaviour and so the patient may present with a similar syndrome to personality disorder. However, it is usually possible to identify from the history that in neuroses the symptoms are primary and predate the onset of behaviour disturbance, whereas the converse occurs in personality disorder. The main points of distinction are shown in Table 6.1.

Another difficulty is separating neuroses from stress reactions. The disorder is described as a neurosis only if the reaction is unusual or

Table 6.1

Main Differences Between Neurosis and Personality Disorder

Neurosis	Personality disorder
Usually short-lived	Persistent through most of adult life
Environmental precipitants common	Fluctuates in response to environmental factors but shows no fundamental change
Presents primarily as symptoms with secondary effects on behaviour	Presents primarily as impairment of personal or social adjustment
Definite change in symptomatology and function in history of disorder	Little or no evidence of change in symptomatology in history of disorder

excessive, so that it is out of keeping with the situation in which it arises. If most people would suffer similar symptoms in that situation, it can be called normal if the symptoms are mild or a stress reaction if they are severe.

To illustrate the overlap between stress or adjustment reactions, neuroses and personality disorders the three diagnostic categories will be described together in each sub-group. Most neuroses have a 'linked' personality disorder which displays somewhat similar symptoms, although some stand alone (Table 6.2).

ANXIETY

Anxiety Neurosis

Anxiety neuroses (or anxiety states) are conditions in which the physical (somatic) and mental (psychic) symptoms of anxiety are the dominant clinical symptoms. If they occur in response to a real threat (such as a threatening telephone call or sudden illness in a close relative) they can be regarded as normal anxiety or a short-lived

Table 6.2

Classification of Neurosis and Personality Disorder

Neurotic disorder	Personality type or personality disorder
Anxiety neurosis (state anxiety)	Anxious personality (trait anxiety)
Phobic neurosis	—
Hysteria	Histrionic personality Asthenic personality
Obsessional neurosis	Anankastic personality
Depressive neurosis	Cyclothymic personality
Hypochondriacal neurosis	Hypochondriacal personality disorder
Depersonalisation syndrome	—
—	Schizoid personality disorder
—	Antisocial personality disorder

response to stress, but if they occur in response to imagined threat only (e.g. going out into the garden) the anxiety is pathological. Anxiety states present in two forms: (i) a more or less continuous state of anxiety which fluctuates to some extent depending on environmental factors, or (ii) sudden unpredictable attacks of anxiety which take the patient quite unawares and are usually accompanied by severe bodily symptoms (Table 6.3). These are called panic attacks. The bodily symptoms may so dominate the clinical picture that the patient feels he must have an organic illness and seeks investigation accordingly.

Because anxiety is one of the easiest emotions to identify, the diagnosis of anxiety state is often over-used by newcomers to psychiatry. It is important to realise that any unpleasant mental event is likely to produce some anxiety and this may be the only manifestation present on the surface. For the diagnosis of anxiety neurosis the pathological symptoms have to be the dominant clinical feature both in terms of severity and duration of symptoms. The most common differential diagnosis is minor depressive illness.

Anxious Personality

Anxiety is a basic drive as well as an emotion and is therefore of biological value. In many ways, those who are anxiety prone have a biological advantage over those who are not, because they take risks less frequently and tend to anticipate the worst. For this reason anxious personalities are not normally described as anxious personality disorders. Such personalities have a lifelong tendency to anxiety when placed under mild stress, sometimes called 'trait' anxiety. This is different from the anxious patient in, for example, a panic attack who exemplifies 'state' anxiety. It is well established that those with high trait anxiety tend to have many more attacks of anxiety neurosis than others of calmer personality. It is therefore difficult to make a distinction between chronic

Table 6.3

Symptoms of Anxiety

Physical	Mental
Muscle tension	Awareness of threat
Tremor	Irritability
Palpitations	Mental tension and worry
Stomach churning	Difficulty in concentration
Diarrhoea	Distractability
Sweating	Intolerance to noise
Nausea	Inability to relax
Dizziness	
Difficulty in breathing	

anxiety neurosis and repeated attacks of anxiety occurring in an anxious personality.

Phobic Neurosis (Phobic Anxiety States)

Phobic anxiety used to be classified with the anxiety neuroses but in recent years their differences (Table 6.4) have become emphasised to a greater extent because they have important implications for treatment. Phobic anxiety is irrational situational anxiety; it is clearly triggered by a single stimulus or set of stimuli which are predictable, and which normally cause no concern to others. The subject tends to use avoidance as a means of coping with the fear. If the fear is a simple one of a single uncommon object such as a large spider, it is comparatively easy to re-order one's

Table 6.4

Differences Between Phobic and Anxiety States

Phobic neurosis	Anxiety neurosis
Anxiety is situational	Anxiety is free-floating
Anxiety predictable	Anxiety unpredictable
Avoidance a common coping stratagem	Avoidance not used

life so that spiders are generally avoided. However, if the phobia is a more handicapping one such as agoraphobia, which literally means fear of the market place and therefore includes open spaces, crowded streets, tall buildings and the feeling of being closed in without a means of escape, it is impossible to avoid all these situations without serious social handicap.

In classifying phobias it is important to separate minor fears that produce little handicap from those that seriously disrupt normal life (Table 6.5). The minor fears are highly specific, of dogs or other animals, thunder and lightning, heights or insects and there are few people that have never had any of them at some point in their lives. Not all these fears are necessarily irrational; so-called snake phobia is a dubious inclusion, as about half the population have such a phobia it probably has biological value. These phobias tend to begin in childhood and, although they usually disappear during development, in some people they persist throughout adult life, and may rarely become severe enough to disrupt normal life. The two main groups of phobias that present to psychiatrists are agoraphobia and social phobia.

Agoraphobia

This is the most common serious phobia; it effects women three times more commonly than men and usually begins in early adult life. In its most severe form it leads to the syndrome of the 'housebound housewife' in which the sufferer becomes literally confined to the home because of acute anxiety whenever she steps outside the confines of the building. Agoraphobics characteristically experience discomfort in buses, trains, shops, cinemas, etc., situations which they tend to avoid, although they may be able to enter them if accompanied by spouse, relative or friend. Many agoraphobics suffer their symptoms for years and their handicap leads to major changes in adjustment for the whole family. A proportion of agoraphobics also have personality disorder, often of the passive-dependent type.

Social phobia

This is about twice as common in women than men. There are fears of social situations, particularly formal ones such as eating in public or ceremonies such as weddings or funerals, in which the underlying fear is often that of ridicule or of doing something foolish. Like agoraphobia it tends to begin in early adult life and is frequent as a temporary phenomenon during adjustment from adolescence to adulthood.

Another group of phobias is often described – illness phobia. This describes an irrational fear of bodily ill-health and overlaps considerably with hypochondriacal and obsessional neuroses. Because this type of phobia is not situational and avoidance is not possible it is not described further here.

Table 6.5

Classification of Phobias

	Monosymptomatic	Agoraphobia	Social phobia
Age of onset	In childhood	Early adult life	Adult life
Feared object	Animals, insects, thunder, heights, etc. (very specific)	Open spaces, crowded places, tall buildings, main roads, public transport (vaguely specific)	Formal social occasions, eating in public, talking in social gatherings (fairly specific)
Prevalence	6%	0·8%	0·5%

HYSTERIA

Hysterical Neurosis

Hysteria differs from other neurotic disorders in that insight is usually lacking and the clinical features can mimic a wide range of psychiatric and organic states. It is a difficult disorder to diagnose because its key feature is unconscious motivation, something that can never be open to experimental proof. The patient finds himself unable to consciously accept the implications of certain emotionally charged events and reacts by 'splitting off' the unpleasant part of the unconscious. This phenomenon is known as 'dissociation' and is often followed by 'conversion' of the symptom into a bodily complaint, such as paralysis, blindness, or apparent fits. Such patients are usually investigated for organic causes before the diagnosis of hysteria can be seriously considered.

In dissociative hysteria the patient suppresses the thought or memory of unpleasant events and pretends that they have not occurred. Hysterical amnesia may be total (global) or selective for the unacceptable event (e.g. over the period of the death of a close relative). Because the symptoms are said to be unconsciously motivated, the condition must be separated from malingering, in which symptoms are simulated consciously for a specific end. There is often symbolic significance in the conversion symptom or type of dissociation which explains the reason for it (e.g. writer's cramp in a student just before an examination).

The status of hysteria as a diagnostic entity is disputed and some claim that, although hysterical symptoms can occur, they do so in the setting of other psychiatric disorder and that a diagnosis of hysteria alone should not be made. Many patients diagnosed as hysterical develop other illness over time and it is right to regard the diagnosis as only a provisional one.

Histrionic and Asthenic Personalities (Passive-dependent Personality Disorder)

In common language 'hysteria' describes one aspect of the behaviour of the histrionic personality, an exaggerated display of emotion that is out of keeping with its setting. Although there is apparent emotional overstatement, there is a superficiality or shallowness of feeling that suggests an absence of fundamental emotion and is illustrated by the fickleness with which one intense emotion dramatically succeeds another. This behaviour has an element of acting in it, as though the subject was a performer always playing to an audience, trying to create an appropriately fashioned role. All the person's actions seem to be done more for their effect on others than for any independent motive. This need to make a good impression is thought to imply a fundamental insecurity, as is the need to be constantly noticed and be a focus of attention. Manipulation of others to achieve goals, childish egocentricity and undue dependence on others are also characteristic of histrionic personality.

Many have criticised the concept of histrionic personality and the author agrees with those who think that it should not be regarded as a personality disorder in itself. Some of the so-called abnormalities of histrionic personality are feminine characteristics that are often admired and lead to better social adjustment rather than handicap. It is not surprising that most people diagnosed as suffering from histrionic personality disorder are women and that those who most use the term are men. Indeed, histrionic personality has been briefly described as man's description of woman, which only in a misogynist world could be considered abnormal.

The asthenic personality is a more obvious disorder. People with asthenic personalities are often described as inadequate, an adjective which is itself inadequate for it has emotional overtones in suggesting that 'adequacy' can be achieved by greater effort. Asthenic personalities have few reserves of resources; when an unusual challenge is present they cannot draw on their experience to find ways of overcoming them and need to turn to outside help. They are always in danger of being swamped by events that they seem powerless to influence or control. Those who are handicapped through physical infirmity or intellectual impairment are not included in this group.

Asthenic personalities usually realise their limitations and use friends, relatives or altruistic agencies for 'first-aid'. They therefore become dependent on people or organisations, be they spouses, charities or government departments. A common reaction from uninformed outside observers is to regard such people as 'spongers' or 'parasites' and to make frequent reference to the pulling up of socks when approached for remedies. Unfortunately the true asthenic personality does not respond to any blandishments and only becomes less resourceful when criticised. It is very common to have additional neurotic symptoms, particularly anxiety and depression in response to adverse pressures, but the abnormal personality remains the prime disturbance.

Because some histrionic personalities are dependent and manipulative because of a real need for support, it is best to combine them with the asthenic personality in a single category, passive-dependent personality disorder. This emphasises the two main factors that lead to social maladjustment: inability to respond to stimuli that demand change, and the need for constant support.

Another condition, named Briquet's syndrome after the French physician who first described it, overlaps with hysteria and passive-dependent personality disorder (and also with hypochondriasis and anxiety states). This has recently become popularised in the United States and describes a syndrome occurring almost exclusively in women in which there are multiple somatic complaints which have no demonstrable organic basis, usually beginning in early adult life and leading to frequent medical consultations. The complaints can be viewed as conversion symptoms but their recurrent nature and the constant need for advice is suggestive of personality disorder.

OBSESSIVE-COMPULSIVE DISORDERS

Obsessional Neurosis

Obsessional neurosis is one of the less common neuroses, accounting for some 2% of referrals to psychiatrists with a prevalence in the population of about 1 in 1000. Obsessional symptoms of short duration are experienced by ten times as many people, often in the course of other psychiatric illness. The key features of an obsessional symptom are: (i) a subjective feeling of compulsion to carry out an act or a thought, (ii) the recognition that the act or thought is pointless or absurd, and (iii) subjective resistance to carrying out the act (ritual) or thought (rumination). The first two characteristics are usually regarded as essential in defining a symptom as obsessional, whereas the third is sometimes lacking. The importance of remembering these features is that, if only the repetitive aspects of the obsessional behaviour are considered, many other non-obsessional disorders such as stereotyped movements in schizophrenia and the repetitive worrying of anxiety would be wrongly regarded as obsessional.

Obsessional neurosis is often separated into obsessive-compulsive neurosis (more appropriately obsessional ritual neurosis), in which rituals predominate, and obsessional ruminative neurosis, in which ruminations are the main factor. It is common to have both ruminations and rituals present together. In obsessional neurosis the symptoms become almost continuous and constantly intrude into consciousness, causing inefficiency and useless pre-occupations. Thus, a housewife will spend the whole day arranging glass ornaments on a mantelpiece so that the light reflects from each in a certain way, and she becomes extremely anxious and distressed if this ritual is prevented or foreshortened. There is a constant need to check that the acts have been done correctly, but no amount of reassurance can remove the small amount of doubt that remains. The French term 'folie de doute' exemplifies this uncertainty of obsessional neurosis. Fears of contamination are also common in the condition. The patient who suspects that he might have been contaminated washes all the articles that he could have touched, then doubts whether his efforts have been successful and washes them all again, extending to new ones that he may have touched in passing. He continues on a cleaning ritual that would make a detergent salesman feel proud. However, just as 'whiter than white' has no end-point where the customer can feel satisfied, the exhausted obsessional can never be certain that his activities have been successful in preventing contamination. Many rituals are derived from superstitions, such as repetitive actions done a certain number of times, with the need to go back to the beginning if interrupted. Just as superstitious behaviour is alleged to ward off evil happenings, the obsessional hopes his rituals will prevent some terrible tragedy.

Obsessional neuroses often last for many years and in such cases are resistant to therapy. Obsessional symptoms occurring in the course of other illnesses have a different course and disappear rapidly with resolution of the illness. The most common differential diagnoses are depressive illness with secondary obsessions, phobic and anxiety states, and hypochondriacal neuroses. Illness phobias, such as fear of cancer or tuberculosis, are midway between obsessions and phobias as, although they are not fully regarded as abnormal (even after a host of normal investigations and examinations) they demonstrate 'folie de doute' and lead to constant ruminations.

Obsessional Personality

The personality disorder linked with obsessional neurosis, the obsessional or anankastic personality disorder, is often confused with obsessional symptoms. In lay use, the word 'obsessional' describes a pre-occupation with order and routine, associated with rigidity and reluctance to change. These features may be found in obsessional neurosis because many such patients have anankastic personality disorder, but they are not features of obsessional neurosis itself. The adjective 'anankastic' is used to describe this personality disorder because, although anankastic is merely derived from a Greek word meaning compulsion, it avoids the use of 'obsessional' and reduces confusion. The main qualities that distinguish the rigid, conforming behaviour of the anankastic personality disorder (often described as typical civil servant behaviour by those who do not like civil servants) from obsessional symptoms is that there is no subjective resistance to the behaviour and it is not considered pointless. Indeed, the opposite view is firmly held, in that the anankast believes that if the rest of the world was as efficient and as well organised as him everything would run more smoothly. Although a high proportion of obsessional neurotics have anankastic personalities, only a minority of anankastic personalities have other psychiatric illness, as the personality disorder is much more common than the neurosis. Under the stress of imposed change the handicap of their rigidity becomes apparent and they are much more likely to fall ill with depression than with obsessional illness.

DEPRESSIVE NEUROSIS AND CYCLOTHYMIC PERSONALITY DISORDER

These have already been discussed in the previous chapter on affective disorders. Depressive neurosis (or minor depressive illness) is the most common of the neuroses, exceeding the total of all the others. Cyclothymic personality disorder describes a lifelong tendency to mood swings that can lead to social maladjustment if they are severe. Because these mood swings may be so marked that the subject demonstrates signs of manic-depressive illness, they are more appropriately dealt with as affective rather than personality disorders.

DEPERSONALISATION SYNDROME

Depersonalisation and derealisation are occasionally found as symptoms in other psychiatric disorders and in normal subjects under special conditions (e.g. after sleep deprivation). They also occur as a prodromal feature in temporal lobe epilepsy. Patients find it difficult to describe the symptoms and often feel embarrassed, because their experience may be misconstrued as evidence of more serious psychiatric illness. In simple terms, depersonalisation is a feeling of unfamiliarity or detachment about the self, whereas derealisation is the same feeling about other people and environments. In describing this feeling both doctors and patients tend to use words such as 'unreal' or 'dream-like', but these are not quite appropriate because the person realises the self and things about him are real but not quite right in a way that is very difficult to describe. It is a more negative feeling than a positive one; an aspect of normal perception is removed and the person recognises the loss.

Depersonalisation and derealisation most commonly occur as symptoms in phobic and anxiety states, and in depression. Depersonalisation seems to be a form of physiological 'cut-off' against extreme anxiety, in that the depersonalised patient has lowered physiological arousal and is protected from the psychic distress of panic attacks. Depersonalisation therefore often occurs

at the height of an anxiety attack and disappears again as the attack is resolving. In severe depressive illness depersonalisation is often present, although it may sometimes be mistaken for nihilistic delusions.

There is a rare disorder, primary depersonalisation syndrome, in which depersonalisation and/or derealisation occur as the sole psychiatric symptom. It usually begins in early adult life and as the change is a sudden one it is indelibly etched in the memory. The condition may be short-lived or may last for years. The sufferer does not outwardly seem distressed and can lead a normal life, but he is constantly aware that he is missing something of the flavour of life, that he is not fully involved.

HYPOCHONDRIASIS

Hypochondriasis includes excessive pre-occupation over health and feelings of imagined illness. It is a frequent symptom in psychiatric disorders. Hypochondriacal delusions are often found in severe depressive illness and in schizophrenia. Hypochondriacal concern over symptoms is common in anxiety states, when the somatic symptoms may be interpreted as symptoms of illness, and mention has already been made of hypochondriasis in Briquet's syndrome, obsessional neurosis and 'illness phobia'. The rare Munchausen syndrome, in which the patient presents with simulated symptoms of acute medical or surgical emergencies in order to gain admission to hospital and have surgical procedures performed, is also sometimes regarded as having a hypochondriacal aspect.

When all the conditions responsible for secondary hypochondriasis have been excluded, there remains a small core of primary hypochondriacal neuroses. These patients are convinced that they have organic illness despite all evidence to the contrary, and they have no symptoms of other psychiatric illness. They frequently present to physicians rather than psychiatrists and are often described as having 'functional disorders'. The reasons why some patients present in this way are far from clear, but presenting with physical symptoms is a socially acceptable form of 'illness behaviour'. Many of these patients are hypersensitive to small changes in their bodily functions and in magnifying them out of all proportion they mistakenly assume organic illness must be present.

When such hypochondriacal symptoms occur in someone whose premorbid personality was relatively stable and without hypochondriacal features, it is best to regard the condition as hypochondriacal neurosis. If, however, the person has been excessively concerned about his health throughout life and has always felt that he had a severe illness at the first sign of ill-health, it is more appropriate to regard him as suffering from hypochondriacal personality disorder.

Neither of these terms should be used too readily because they imply resistance to treatment and a relatively poor outcome.

SCHIZOID PERSONALITY DISORDER

A schizoid personality disorder has no neurotic counterpart, although it does have links with schizophrenic illness. Many patients with schizoid personality disorders do not develop schizophrenia or any other psychiatric illness, but there is some overlap between the clinical features of the two conditions. Schizoid individuals are isolated, aloof people who find it difficult to make close relationships with others and are often regarded as cold and detached. Because of these difficulties they seldom achieve any close personal relationships and become eccentric in their habits and beliefs. Their oddness shows itself to others and they then become more isolated. Their introversion is sometimes so marked that they are completely bound up in a fantasy world of their own. In the past many people with schizoid personalities opted out of society and became vagrants or hermits. This lifestyle was not inappropriate for them, for it allowed them to express their eccentricity and fantasies without causing any concern to others. Some schizoid personalities also show excessive suspiciousness and rigidity, when they are described as paranoid personalities. Such people are excessively pre-occupied with their rights and will go to great lengths to defend them. They are sensitive to criticism and rapidly take offence.

ANTISOCIAL (SOCIOPATHIC) PERSONALITY DISORDER

This important group of personality disorders includes a wide range of abnormalities that fundamentally cause offence to society. Involvement with the forces of law and order is therefore common and many such patients come to psychiatric attention through the courts. The term 'psychopathy' (p.132) is often used to describe this group but it is not preferred here, because it has been distorted and devalued by indiscriminate use.

The person with an antisocial personality disorder normally has a history of such behaviour from an early age. Truancy, childhood aggression and petty offences are common and there is often a history of emotional deprivation, with parental separation and frequent disruptions in family life, often with supervision outside the family such as in children's homes or by foster parents. The inconsistencies in this upbringing do not allow the child to develop a stable set of values or lifestyle. In adult life such people remain emotionally immature and irresponsible. They lack moral sense and feel little guilt, so that they can readily commit offences for immediate gain.

Such personality disorders are sometimes subdivided into those who are emotionally hot-tempered and impulsive but who regret their actions afterwards (explosive personality disorder) and those who are colder and more calculating, with little feeling for their fellow men, and who can become dangerous criminals because of their innate callousness and lack of respect for life. Aggression is common in both groups but it is potentially much more serious in the second. Antisocial personality disorder is diagnosed many more times frequently in men than in women for reasons which may be similar to the explanation of female preponderance of histrionic personality disorder.

DIFFERENTIAL DIAGNOSIS

Personality disorder is not easy to diagnose and to some extent it is used as a term of criticism or therapeutic impotence. Its prevalence is between 1 and 2% in the population, with the antisocial and passive-dependent groups providing two-thirds of the total. Because personality disorder cannot be diagnosed by simple examination of the mental state, it is often not considered as a possible diagnosis until after a patient has failed to respond to treatment. This in itself is not an adequate reason for diagnosing personality disorder and it is always wise to consider this possibility at the outset. It can often be suspected from the history but confirmation is needed through interview with a close relative or other informant of the patient because they are best placed to describe any adverse social impact of the personality.

Both neurosis and personality disorder can co-exist and it is quite appropriate to make two diagnoses, one of the personality and the other of mental illness. However, it is often important to decide whether the presenting problem is primarily due to neurosis or personality disorder and the scheme outlined in Fig. 6.1 is designed to achieve this. It can only be followed after both patient and informant have been interviewed, so that the duration and intensity of the symptoms as well as the extent of personal maladjustment has been assessed.

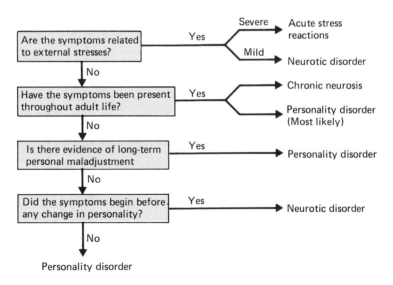

Fig. 6.1 *The separation of stress reactions, neurosis and personality disorder.*

TREATMENT OF NEUROSES

There is no common factor governing the treatment of neuroses, and the indications for treatment are less clear-cut than in the functional psychoses. It is therefore best to discuss the value of each type of therapy in individual neurotic categories.

Psychotherapy

Psychotherapy is discussed in Chapter 12. Since psychoanalytic treatment was originally devised for the treatment of hysteria, dynamic psychotherapy might seem the treatment of choice for that disorder. A more rapid procedure, often effective in the removal of a particular symptom, is abreaction, the reliving of a highly traumatic experience that has been consciously suppressed. Abreaction is facilitated by the intravenous administration of small doses of a benzodiazepine or a barbiturate, which decrease cortical inhibition and enable expression of the suppressed material. Abreaction may also be used with some forms of minor depressive disorder as an aid to 'working-through' loss.

Dynamic psychotherapy may be used in severe anxiety and hypochondriacal neuroses and the depersonalisation syndrome. In less severe forms of neurosis, including those that have become chronic, supportive psychotherapy may be of considerable value.

Behaviour Therapy

Behaviour therapy is also discussed in Chapter 12, where the treatment of agoraphobia is considered. A similar form of treatment can be applied to social phobia. Behaviour therapy has its highest rates of success in the treatment of monosymptomatic phobias.

Extinction of maladaptive behaviour patterns is also used in treating obsessional neurosis. The obsessional ritual, as noted earlier, is an anxiety relieving activity which protects the patient from alleged calamity. If the rituals are prevented, anxiety levels rise but the calamity does not occur, so that the obsession is relieved. More complex behavioural techniques have been devised to deal with individual obsessional symptoms.

Relaxation techniques can be considered along with behaviour therapy although they are not derived from learning theory; they involve relaxation by conscious effort through relaxation of voluntary muscles and internal self-instruction to be calm. They are essential to yoga, transcendental meditation and similar philosophical therapies, but can also be practised alone. They are often helpful in patients with trait anxiety.

Pharmacological Treatment (see Chapter 13)

Drugs are also widely used in the treatment of neuroses, although sometimes inappropriately. It is best to consider them as adjuncts to other treatments rather than sole therapy. Benzodiazepines are appropriate for short-term or intermittent treatment of phobias and anxiety, particularly when the anxiety becomes so intense that normal function is impossible. Neuroleptic drugs in low dosage may also be useful, particularly as they do not give rise to any pharmacological dependence. Beta-blockers (such as propranolol) may give relief when physical symptoms of anxiety are prominent. In severe cases of phobic anxiety, and to a lesser extent in anxiety and hypochondriacal neuroses, tricyclic antidepressants (such as clomipramine) or monoamine oxidase inhibitors (MAOIs) (such as phenelzine) may be used. The evidence suggests that both groups of drugs are effective but that MAOIs are slightly superior. In obsessional neurosis clomipramine is often used and is effective in some cases; it is difficult to know if this is because it is treating depressive aspects of the neurosis or the obsessional symptoms directly.

There is no satisfactory treatment of the depersonalisation syndrome although some psychostimulant drugs can artificially bring back reality. The effect is usually transient. Their risk of dependence generally precludes their use. A summary of the treatment of the neuroses is shown in Table 6.6.

TREATMENT OF PERSONALITY DISORDER

Unfortunately there is no satisfactory treatment for personality disorder. The secondary symptomatology can be treated in the same way as in neurotic disorders but the primary problem, the personality, remains. Indeed, many would view the development of a successful treatment for personality disorder with alarm because of social and political implications for normal personality. The aim in management is to place the patient in a setting where his deviant personality traits have the least impact. Often these traits can be put to positive use, so the anankastic personality will be an excellent quality controller on an assembly line where he is checking the final product, or a schizoid personality can be sent by his employer on long assignments with only himself for company. Most of the suitable lifestyles for people with personality disorders are a little unusual but they can be very productive. Although attempts have been made to modify behaviour in antisocial personality disorder by extension of principles based on the therapeutic community the evidence for success is scanty. However, there is some evidence that antisocial personality disorders improve with the passage of time and may resolve entirely in middle age.

Table 6.6

Treatment of Neuroses (the preferred treatment for each disorder is given in italics)

Neurosis	Psychotherapy	Behaviour therapy	Drug therapy
Anxiety	Supportive	*Relaxation techniques*	Benzodiazepines
Hysteria	*Interpretive* (abreaction)	Operant conditioning	Not appropriate
Phobic	Interpretive	*Desensitisation*	Benzodiazepines MAOIs
		Exposure in vivo	Clomipramine
Obsessional	Supportive	Techniques to control different symptoms	Clomipramine
Hypochondriacal	*Supportive*	Relaxation techniques	Antidepressant drugs
Depersonalisation	Interpretive	Not appropriate	Psychostimulants (but rarely appropriate)

7

The Psychiatry of Old Age

INTRODUCTION

The psychiatry of old age (psychogeriatrics) is concerned with all types of mental illness, functional and organic, which occur in late life. Its claim to be considered as a sub-specialty within psychiatry is founded not only upon the special medical and service needs of older people, but also upon clinical differences of emphasis. The elderly suffer essentially from the same disorders as younger patients, but these disorders tend to manifest themselves in particular ways and to require a different approach towards assessment and management.

EPIDEMIOLOGY

The elderly are consumers on a large scale of health-care resources, not only because they are a vulnerable group, but also because life expectancy has significantly increased during their lifetime. In 1900 only 5% of the total population was over 65 years old; at the beginning of the 1980s the proportion is about 15% (Fig. 7.1). Psychiatric morbidity in this age group is high, mainly due to dementia and depression. Some 6 to 10% of the population over 65 suffers from dementia (chronic organic psychosyndrome), a half of that proportion severely. This means that there are about

650 000 affected individuals in the United Kingdom. Community surveys have shown that only a minority (at best one in five) of these unfortunate people are receiving hospital care. The majority are at home, frequently in extremely squalid and/or precarious conditions.

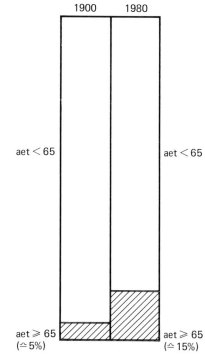

Fig. 7.1 *Proportionate growth in the elderly population since 1900.*

64

The elderly are more susceptible than younger people to affective disorder. Hospital first admission rates for depression, an indication of the most serious cases, reach a peak in the sixth and seventh decades of life, and begin to fall steeply only well into the eighth. As with dementia, morbidity in the community is high. Moreover, as many as two-thirds of those with significant, yet potentially treatable, depressive symptoms may be unknown to their family doctor.

PRINCIPLES OF ASSESSMENT

Psychiatric patients of all ages are often unable to give a coherent history by virtue of their mental disorder, but this is particularly true of elderly patients. It may therefore be necessary to seek out actively other more reliable informants, such as relatives, friends and neighbours. The active pursuit of reliable informants can make excessive demands on medical time, so that the involvement of colleagues from other disciplines, such as social workers, nurses and care assistants, in the assessment/diagnostic process is of major importance. Whether this team is based on a hospital or health centre its members should be mobile and willing to undertake home assessment. This can assist not only in arriving at a diagnosis, but also give vital information on the patient's ability to function within his/her normal environment. Home assessment is not required in every case, but is preferable in many. If the patient is to be admitted to hospital there are great advantages in a joint assessment unit with the geriatric team, because the concurrence of mental and physical disorders in the elderly is common. Even if such units do not exist in particular areas, close cooperation between psychiatrist and physician in assessment and management should always be possible.

PRINCIPLES OF MANAGEMENT

Where to treat

The decision where to treat (hospital or community) can be crucial. For instance, a patient who is coping, albeit precariously, at home can experience such disorientation on admission to hospital that the mental disorder worsens and the ability to cope, even with the most basic self-care, disappears. It may therefore be preferable to opt for day hospital or similar facilities, where feasible, rather than removal from a familiar environment.

Drugs

Medication for elderly out-patients can present special problems of compliance. Memory disturbance short of frank dementia may lead to erratic drug taking, either inadequate or excessive. Severely agitated patients can attribute worsening depressive symptoms to their medication itself and stop taking it. Thus, unobtrusive supervision by a relative, district nurse or other suitable person is often helpful.

The elderly are particularly sensitive to unwanted effects of drugs. As a rule of thumb lower initial doses, and lower therapeutic doses achieved gradually over longer periods are required. Prescription of a variety of drugs is to be avoided, especially where additional medication is prescribed for physical disorders. A large array of tablets to be taken at different times of the day can be very baffling for an elderly person and may exacerbate or even precipitate some mental disorders.

Psychotherapy

Psychotherapy with older patients is usually of a simpler kind, avoiding complex psychodynamic interpretations based on early experiences, focusing instead upon an empathic relationship between patient and therapist. Long-term supportive psychotherapy in chronic depression and other functional disorders, even permitting indefinite dependence on the therapist, can contribute greatly to keeping patients out of hospital and at home. Group therapy can also be valuable. Here, too, there is less concern with depth psychology than with a shared approach to such mutual problems as widowhood, loneliness and financial insecurity.

Hospitalisation

When patients are admitted to hospital greater attention has to be paid to their physical needs, including bowel and bladder function. For example, the anticholinergic effects of tricyclic antidepressants can cause or aggravate constipation and prostatism; urinary retention can occur; a trivial urinary tract infection can exacerbate dementia; insomnia may be due to orthopnoea and therefore better treated with diuretics in the morning than hypnotics at night.

The occupational therapist has a vital role to play together with the nursing staff in the maintenance of simple functions such as dressing, self-care and the handling of everyday finances which most of us take for granted, but which can be severely eroded by mental disorder and the dependent setting of hospital. Older patients adapt with difficulty to hospitalisation; once settled they can experience difficulty in re-adapting to life at home. Thus, a flexible, longitudinal approach to discharge is preferable, with several trial periods at home of increasing duration before final separation from hospital.

AFFECTIVE DISORDER

Depressive Illness

Aetiology

The elderly suffer from both manic and depressive illness, although the latter is by far the commoner. Not only are older people more susceptible to depression, but also successful suicide rates, especially in men, increase with age. The reasons for this vulnerability to serious depression are partly environmental and partly constitutional.

Common sense dictates that old age is a period of loss: loss of social status, employment, physical capacity and financial security, all enhancing loss of self-esteem. Worse still, spouse and friends are lost through bereavement, while children move away from home and form emotional attachments elsewhere. Illness and bereavement serve as unpleasant reminders of mortality.

Genetic studies have indicated that depressive illness emerging for the first time in old age is less likely than that of earlier onset to be associated with a family history of affective disorder. Furthermore, late onset depression shows no tendency to be manifested in particularly vulnerable personalities.

Cerebrovascular disease and depression in old people co-exist more frequently than by chance, but the organic disorder probably precipitates the functional one in susceptible individuals. Recent neurophysiological research has yielded data suggesting that the emergence of depression in old age may be facilitated by an ageing process in the CNS. Its precise nature is unclear, but it is unrelated to cerebrovascular disease. Furthermore, elderly depressed patients show a higher mortality from general causes than the age-matched normal population.

Clinical picture

Depressive symptoms are not unique to any age, but depression in late life is more commonly characterised by anxiety and agitation than by psychomotor retardation. Typically the patient is restless, tearful and repeatedly importunes for reassurance. Bizarre histrionic behaviour out of keeping with the premorbid personality may be observed. Delusional ideas are common, sometimes with a basis in reality, e.g. understandable financial problems leading to delusions of impoverishment, at other times fantastic, e.g. nihilistic beliefs that the whole or part of the body no longer exists. At an age of vulnerability to physical illness it is not surprising that hypochondriacal preoccupations and delusions are also common.

Some patients may not show any obvious disorder of mood, but exhibit hypochondriacal symptoms with or without biological disturbances, such as insomnia and anorexia. This is called 'masked depression', and responds well to antidepressant treatment. Other patients perform so poorly on cognitive testing that they appear to be demented. Depressive symptoms have usually appeared before the onset of cognitive impairment, but may be discovered only by a careful history from a reliable informant. This phenomenon of apparent cognitive failure is termed 'depressive pseudodementia'. A pseudodemented patient is more likely to respond to pertinent questions with 'I don't know', whereas a truly demented person may give a confabulated answer. It is vitally important to differentiate pseudo- from true dementia in order that a treatable illness is not missed. Where diagnostic doubt remains no harm is done by a trial of antidepressant treatment. Similar action can be taken in the few cases where it is difficult to differentiate depression from late paraphrenia (schizophrenia-like illness – see below), because of the prominence of bizarre delusions. These often have a basis in guilt if they are depressive, e.g. the patient believes he/she is pursued by the police because of some minor misdemeanour in the past or a more serious but imagined crime. As always a careful history searching for evidence of depressive symptoms will help to elucidate the majority of cases.

Treatment

Old people respond well to all physical treatments, but their susceptibility to unwanted effects means that lower doses of drugs are used. For example, a healthy young adult may start with 75 mg amitriptyline daily rising to 150–200 mg over one week, whereas an elderly patient starts with 25 mg daily rising to 50–100 mg over two weeks. Sometimes the therapeutic dose is lower than this. Tricyclic antidepressants such as amitriptyline and imipramine are preferred to tetracyclic preparations, not least because the tricyclics are very much cheaper and no less effective. However, concurrent cardiac, prostatic or Parkinson's disease may call for the costlier, but less anticholinergic, tetracyclics such as mianserin in an initial dose of 10 mg at night, increasing to 40–60 mg over two weeks. Electroconvulsive therapy (ECT) is well tolerated and is particularly effective for the psychotic (deluded) patient. As ECT is administered in controlled conditions, it can be considerably safer than a course of drugs in a frail old person. Furthermore, clinical improvement often occurs earlier than with drugs.

Outcome

Although response to antidepressant treatment is good, the relapse rate is high. For this reason, when an antidepressant drug has been prescribed, it should be continued for several months after recovery from a first illness. After subsequent illnesses there is a case for indefinite continuation therapy in low to moderate dosage, which can sometimes obviate long-term hospitalisation.

The older the patient at first onset of depression (especially older than 70) the greater the chance of relapse. Other adverse prognostic factors are organic brain disease, extracerebral physical illness, a senile physique and prolonged uninterrupted depression of two years or more. A small minority of patients require long-term hospital care.

Manic Illness

Manic illness in the elderly is not as rare as was

previously thought. Indeed, mania may manifest itself for the first time in old age after a long latent period following an earlier depressive episode. There may also be an association between coarse brain disease and mania in late life. Clinically a 'mixed affective' picture is characteristic, that is to say manic and depressive symptoms occurring together in the same illness.

Most elderly patients with mania require admission to hospital, principally because their relative frailty exposes them to greater risks. For instance, an old and hyperactive woman is in special danger of falling and sustaining a fractured femur. Treatment with neuroleptic drugs is indicated as it is with younger patients, but usually at a lower dosage. The elderly also respond well to lithium prophylaxis for recurrent mania. Serum lithium levels are kept at the lower end of the therapeutic range, i.e. below 1 mmol/l, because of the risk of impaired renal clearance of lithium. Clearance is reduced in heart and kidney disease, low sodium and fluid intake, and treatment with thiazide diuretics.

Neurosis

Neurotic symptoms are commonly encountered in elderly people. They occur alone or in conjunction with other disorders such as depression and even dementia in its early stages. In this population neurotic symptoms can have been lifelong, or just as commonly arise *de novo* in old age. This fresh emergence of neurosis has often been authoritatively denied, because many patients suffer undetected in the community or, when they do present to doctors, are mistakenly thought to have the physical disorders of which they complain. Personality traits such as anxiety, rigidity, insecurity and a tendency to histrionic, manipulative behaviour are specifically associated with neurotic symptoms in elderly people. Also important are loneliness and physical illness, especially heart disease.

Symptoms are varied and sometimes colourful, ranging through phobic anxiety, hypochondriasis and dissociative hysterical reactions such as paralyses, bizarre gait disturbances and drop attacks. Treatment consists first in the recognition and appropriate management of any underlying functional or organic disorder. Thus, treatment of depression results in resolution of neurotic symptoms. However, if the neurotic disorder is primary, psychotherapy is the principal approach. Even if long-term dependence on the therapist is encouraged, much functional improvement and relief of suffering can be achieved.

LATE PARAPHRENIA

Late paraphrenia is the term used to cover those functional disorders of old age characterised by delusions and hallucinations of a persecutory nature, and which bear varying degrees of resemblance to schizophrenia found in earlier adult life. Approximately 10% of patients over the age of 60 admitted to psychiatric wards suffer from late paraphrenia.

Clinical picture

Three subgroups based on the clinical picture, have been distinguished. The first which has been called 'paranoid hallucinosis' is a condition in which there are circumscribed persecutory, auditory hallucinations. The patient is typically an elderly woman whose only complaint is that she hears the neighbours plotting against her. The second subgroup has been termed 'schizophreniform'. Here delusions are more extensive and may be systematised. Ideas of reference and auditory hallucinations are commonly found. The third subgroup, called 'schizophrenic', is indistinguishable from the condition found in earlier life, with (Schneiderian) first-rank symptoms such as thought interference, delusional perception, and passivity experiences.

Aetiology

With regard to genetic loading late paraphrenia occupies an intermediate position, a family history of schizophrenia being found more commonly than in the normal population, but less frequently than in early onset schizophrenia. A greater preponderance of females to males (about four to one) also contrasts with schizophrenia.

Compared to elderly patients suffering from dementia and affective disorders, those with late paraphrenia show poorer premorbid personality adjustment. Few have made successful marriages, and many remain single having failed or been unwilling to make close personal relationships. However, the relentless social decline towards homelessness and vagrancy, often seen in younger schizophrenics, is not typical of late paraphrenia, where patients may have shown a good work record and social stability right up until the onset of symptoms. A further important aetiological factor is deafness starting in earlier life. Indeed, it is not difficult to understand that worsening hearing loss will exacerbate a tendency to paranoid interpretation in a predisposed individual.

Treatment and outcome

No distinction between the clinical subgroups can be made in respect of aetiology, response to treatment and outcome. These patients respond well to the careful administration of neuroleptic drugs, and a complete remission of symptoms can be expected in at least 50% of cases. Where a complete remission is not achieved sufficient recovery to allow a continuation of or return to an independent existence can be expected in the majority. It is desirable to choose a neuroleptic with a relatively milder antidopaminergic action, such as thioridazine, because of the susceptibility of the elderly to unwanted effects such as Parkinsonism, acute dystonic reactions (e.g. oculogyric crisis) and tardive dyskinesea. In a small minority of severer cases, however, more strongly antidopaminergic preparations such as trifluoperazine or haloperidol may be required. While outcome is generally favourable, relapse most commonly follows the patient's initiative, contrary to medical advice, to stop medication. In most cases treatment should be continued indefinitely.

ORGANIC DISORDERS

Acute Organic Psychosyndromes (Delirium)

Delirium in the elderly is one of the mental disorders most frequently encountered by the medical and surgical resident doctor. It is therefore essential to acquire the ability to recognise and treat the condition. The clinical picture, causation and management are described in Chapter 3 (p.20). Only a few points need to be stressed here. The elderly are the group most vulnerable to acute organic confusion because so many are predisposed to it by underlying chronic brain disease ranging from mild memory impairment to frank dementia. There is, as it were, a loss of functional cerebral reserve. In a previously fit young adult brain, function has to be severely compromised before confusion appears. In the elderly confusion is frequently precipitated or exacerbated by drugs. In an old person with dementia a mild, even subclinical urinary tract infection or slight postoperative fluid and electrolyte imbalance can precipitate clouding of consciousness. Accurate diagnosis is of paramount importance because of the frequent but mistaken assumption that symptoms are due to chronic irreversible brain disease.

Other significant exacerbating or causative factors include varying degrees of sensory deprivation. Delirious states are worse at night because of the absence of visual orientating cues. Similarly, an older person with cataracts, failing vision or blindfolding after an eye operation is permanently 'in the dark'. Defective hearing can also impair orientation. A fluctuating level of consciousness, with or without focal neurological signs should alert suspicion of a subdural haematoma. The elderly differ from younger people in that a subdural haematoma can be precipitated by a trivial injury which might have passed un-noticed several weeks before.

The treatment of delirium is that of the underlying physical disorder, which many elderly patients fail to survive. The management of a delirious patient, who may be trying to pull out a urinary catheter or intravenous line, calls for the highest nursing skill. Calm handling in a side-room away from the bustle of an open ward is desirable. Drip-feed stands, ECG monitors, etc., are likely to increase confusion, so the patient should be surrounded by familiar objects, such as flowers, clocks and photographs of relatives.

Suppression of mental symptoms by medication is to be avoided, if possible, because it can actively hinder recovery from the physical disorder. For example, postoperative pneumonia will not be improved by the use of heavy sedation which impairs the patient's ability to cough up infected sputum. Sometimes, however, sedation has to be given. Injections, other than via existing intravenous lines, are perceived by the confused as an assault and should be avoided. Small oral doses of drugs such as chlormethiazole or promazine can be used instead.

Chronic Organic Psychosyndromes (Dementia)

Types

Dementia of old age is a major epidemic facing

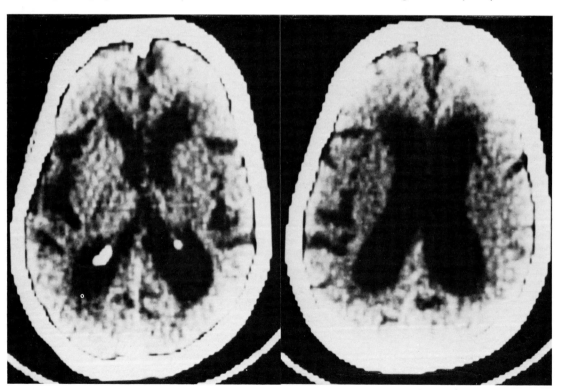

Fig. 7.2 *Computed tomogram (CT scan) of a patient with senile dementia of the Alzheimer type (SDAT) showing ventricular dilatation and sulcal widening.*

developed countries at the end of this century. There are two pathological conditions accounting for the vast majority of cases. First and most common is senile dementia of the Alzheimer type (SDAT), so-called because the histology (senile plaques and neurofibrillary tangles) is identical to the presenile condition described by Alzheimer in 1907 (Fig. 7.2). There is a relationship between the number of plaques in the brain and the degree of clinical impairment.

The second most important cause of dementia in old age is multi-infarct dementia (MID) in which clinical impairment is related to the volume of infarcted brain tissue following cerebral haemorrhage, thrombosis or embolism. Infarcts may be small and diffuse throughout the brain. There is usually but not invariably a history of strokes. Occasionally, when no such history is forthcoming, careful direct questioning reveals that at some time in the past there was a transient manifestation such as drooping of the mouth on one side, or a brief period of acute mental confusion.

A third important cause of dementia is a combination of SDAT and MID, which may produce clinical symptoms with a senile plaque count and volume of cerebral infarction below the individual thresholds required to give either SDAT or MID alone. All other causes of dementia in old age, such as Huntington's chorea, cerebral tumour, myxoedema, Jakob-Creutzfeldt disease, etc., are either uncommon or rare.

Clinical course

Senile dementia of the Alzheimer type and multi-infarct dementia both lead to a fatal outcome, but their clinical development usually differs. The typical course of SDAT begins with insidious memory impairment, evolves into more diffuse higher function deficits, such as dysphasia, dyspraxia, agnosia, impoverishment of thought and emotion as well as more severe memory impairment, and proceeds with a steady deterioration

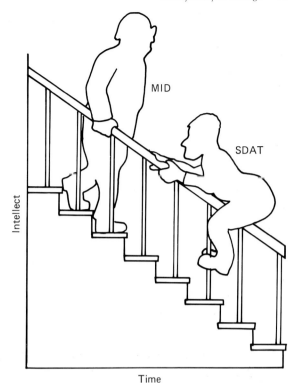

Fig. 7.3 *Diagram illustrating the stepwise clinical deterioration in multi-infarct dementia (MID) compared with the steady decline in senile dementia of the Alzheimer type (SDAT).*

into gross behavioural disturbances such as incontinence of urine and faeces. Patients eventually die of inanition and intercurrent infection, usually pneumonia. In contrast to the steady downhill course of SDAT the natural history of MID is typically that of a stepwise deterioration (Fig. 7.3). There is a stroke followed by intellectual and neurological deficit. Partial recovery may occur without further deterioration until the next cerebrovascular catastrophe. Death is caused by another stroke, intercurrent infection or an unrelated illness. A more detailed account of the clinical manifestations of chronic organic disorders is given in Chapter 3.

Aetiology and prevention

Until recently the aetiology of SDAT has remained a mystery. Senile plaques are found in small numbers in clinically unaffected individuals dying of unrelated diseases. This has led to the hypothesis that SDAT might be a form of abnormal or accelerated ageing. However, at the present time most authorities do not consider this to be the case and regard SDAT as a disease process distinct from biological ageing. Recent research has revived interest in the causation of SDAT with the discovery of a specific deficit of the enzyme choline acetyl transferase in brain areas where the histopathological changes are most marked. A biochemical deficiency of this nature offers a real prospect of specific treatment in the future.

The aetiology of MID is that of atherosclerosis and cerebrovascular disease. Prevention is therefore the primary concern. Elimination or alleviation of risk factors such as hypertension and smoking, and possibly dietary changes, are the measures most likely to reduce the prevalence.

Management

Although no specific treatment for these conditions is yet available much can be done to relieve suffering and even to regain lost ground. Accurate diagnosis with determination of functional cerebral deficits is the first step for the following reasons: acute reversible causes of organic mental confusion are pinpointed and treated; the prognosis can be estimated and plans made for future needs; a systematic approach can be made towards functional deficits.

After diagnosis the present social requirements must be considered. Is it safe to leave the patient at home with gas appliances and open electric fires? If he/she is to remain there, are home-help or meals on wheels required? Could a spouse's burden be relieved by day care (local authority day centre, psychiatric day hospital) or by a planned holiday-relief in-patient admission?

All physical disorders, especially minor ones, which exacerbate the condition are treated. Constipation is relieved; hearing-aids and spectacles are provided; ill-fitting dentures are replaced; night sedation is prescribed for nocturnal rest without daytime stupor. As far as specific cerebral deficits are concerned a negative attitude produces negative results, whereas the more attempted the more achieved. For instance, spatial and temporal disorientation can be improved by constant rehearsal. Dressing dyspraxia may be circumvented by practice and avoidance of difficult items of clothing such as complicated belts and lace-up shoes. Above all maximum use is made of skills and knowledge acquired and practised well before the onset of symptoms. Conversely, activities requiring new learning are kept to a minimum. This is exemplified by the simple but invaluable advice that patients at home should be discouraged from moving house away from a familiar neighbourhood.

A proportion of patients will no longer be able to maintain an independent existence, with or without support, at home. Those with no gross behavioural or physical disorders can be accommodated in local authority residential care. Those more severely impaired require long-term hospital care.

Many of these patients die within a short time of admission. For those who survive longer humane management is not only a moral imperative. The more actively therapeutic and less nihilistic the environment, the more rewarding it is for the staff, who will in turn seek further improvements for patients in their care. The devoted terminal management these patients deserve helps to maintain the dignity which the disease process itself so relentlessly erodes.

CASE ILLUSTRATIONS

Delirium

A woman of 75 with diabetes, myocardial infarction and a Colles' fracture became acutely disturbed, disorientated and said she could see pigeons flying around the (medical) ward. Treatment of the physical disorders alone led to remission of mental symptoms, enabling her to return home.

Depressive Pseudodementia

An accountant of 72 presented with apathy and cognitive impairment. A computed tomogram scan showed some cerebral atrophy. A diagnosis of senile dementia was made. Later his daughter said that intellectual decline had been preceded by anorexia, sleep disturbance and self denigration. Antidepressant treatment resulted in full clinical recovery, although the scan appearances were unchanged.

Masked Depression

A man of 67 'feeling very ill' discharged himself from a medical ward because he was 'no better'. He denied depression ascribing weight loss and insomnia to a physical disorder, 'probably cancer'. Soon readmitted to another hospital convinced of cancer he again threatened to discharge himself. Transferred to a psychiatric ward he recovered after ECT.

Acute on Chronic Organic Psychosyndrome

A demented man of 70 lived with his daughter. He was continent and exhibited no unmanageable behaviour. Over 48 hours he became aggressive and disorientated, especially at night, wandering in the street in his pyjamas. On admission to hospital he was mildly dehydrated with spurious diarrhoea from a faecal impaction, correction of which returned him to his previously stable state.

Late Paraphrenia

A spinster of 78 went to the police station refusing to leave because she had heard neighbours planning to blow up her flat. On admission to hospital she had difficulty grasping questions. She was given a hearing aid and thioridazine was started. Two months later she returned home.

Agitated Depression

A 'straight-laced' widow of 70 became agitated and tearful. She complained of feeling 'desperately ill', asserting it was punishment for 'dirty thoughts'. Amitriptyline was started, but she stopped it because 'it made me worse'. She agreed to ECT believing it would kill her, which she deserved. After ten treatments she was fit to return home.

Dementia – The Value of Premorbid Memory

A demented man of 71 frequently got lost outside his home. His wife said they had recently visited friends in the block where they had lived for 30 years until nine months before. Her husband went missing there, and had been found on the doorstep of their old flat. He had gone to the local shop, purchased tobacco, and returned without difficulty.

8

Suicide and Deliberate Self Harm

SUICIDE

Suicide is studied in psychiatry because death from suicide is the most important cause of the excess mortality of the mentally ill and there are grounds for believing that effective treatment can prevent suicide.

Definition

Suicide as a cause of death can only be decided by a coroner. He reaches this decision after an inquest, where he decides if the evidence proves that the deceased intended death by his actions. The law requires proof and those self inflicted deaths where the evidence falls short of proof are registered as undetermined or accidental deaths. Official statistics underestimate the incidence of suicide by about 30%.

Epidemiology

Four thousand of the 600 000 deaths each year in England and Wales are due to suicide, about 1%. The suicide rate is 8 per 100 000. Suicide is among the ten most important causes of death, but in the young is exceeded by accidents and cancers. The suicide rate is now rising.

Since 1900 the suicide rate has shown variations which point towards some of the causes of suicide (Fig. 8.1). The rate declined in both world wars, as it did in all combatant countries, suggesting that the social cohesion, induced by combining to fight a common enemy, prevents suicide. The rate increased during the great economic depression, as it did in all western countries, suggesting the social and psychological effects of unemployment cause suicide.

From 1963 to 1970 the suicide rate declined from 12 to 7 per 100 000, a fall unique among

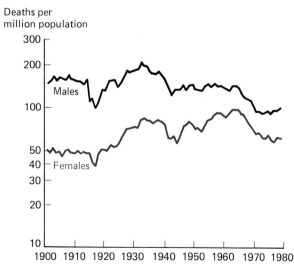

Fig. 8.1 *Suicides: Crude death rates per million living from 1901 to 1978 in England and Wales (male and female).*

European countries. The explanations put forward include economic prosperity and the Samaritan organisation. I believe the removal of carbon monoxide from the town gas supply to have had the strongest influence, with some contribution from the increasingly skilled use of antidepressants by family doctors (and lithium carbonate by psychiatrists). The removal of other dangers from the environment should further reduce suicide, as should better treatment for the mentally ill.

Since 1900 the suicide rate for males has declined and that for females increased, which may reflect the profound changes which have taken place in their social and economic status.

The suicide rate in western countries increases with age, peaking in the 60s for women and the 70s for men (Fig. 8.2). The reverse has been observed in non-western societies, suggesting that the place of the aged in the social structure of a society may have as important an influence as the biological changes of ageing. Men have a suicide rate greater than that of women.

The suicide rate for married people is lower than that for the single, and the widowed and divorced have higher rates than the unmarried. The apparent protective influence of marriage is probably due to more than one cause. The patient with early onset mental illness may be unmarriageable, and later onset mental disorder or alcohol addiction may result in divorce. The death of a spouse may provoke a depressive illness and suicide. The fact that recent bereavement, recent divorce and living alone are all associated with increased risk of suicide suggests that the marital status relationship represents the combined influence of mental illness, recent personal distress and domestic isolation.

Social classes I and V have the highest suicide rates. Social class V at one time had the lowest suicide rate. A change in composition by downward drift of people whose employment has been adversely influenced by mental illness, drink and unstable personality is the likely explanation.

Suicide rates vary across a country. Low rates

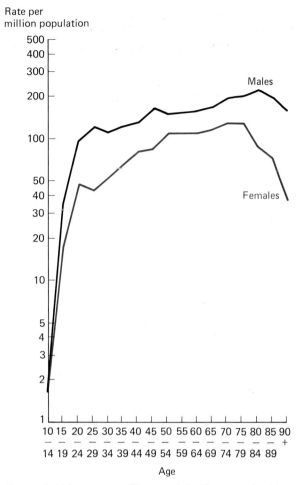

Fig. 8.2 *Suicide rates per million population (by age and sex) in England and Wales; averages for 1976–1978.*

are found in rural areas, higher rates in towns. Within large cities, the highest rates occur in the inner city of lodging houses, bedsitters, and hotels. Lower rates occur in settled working class communities and suburbs. A convincing explanation is the disorganised community produced by a high concentration of 'non-private households' to which are attracted the chronically mentally ill, and those addicted to alcohol and drugs.

The suicide rate has a seasonal rhythm, increasing in early summer. The adverse psychological effect on the unhappy isolate of the increased social activity of spring is one explanation.

Clinical

Mental illness has a high suicide rate and so does alcohol and drug addiction. The suicide rate of patients with schizophrenia, manic depressive psychosis, depressive neurosis, personality disorder, alcohol addiction and 'hard drug' addiction is increased 10–25 times. Fifteen per cent of deaths will eventually be due to suicide compared with 1–2% for the general population.

Death from causes undetermined and from accident are also increased, especially for those addicted to alcohol and drugs.

By combining the suicide mortality rates of mental illnesses and their prevalence the annual expected number of suicides can be estimated and this number approximates to that observed. This calculation suggests that most suicides are mentally ill or addicted to alcohol or drugs at the time they die. Psychiatric studies of consecutive cases of suicide by interviewing those who knew them strongly support this being so.

Depressive illness and alcohol addiction (often present together) account for some 80% of diagnoses. Schizophrenia (5%), addiction to drugs, neuroses and rarer conditions such as anorexia nervosa account for the rest. Five per cent are not diagnosed mentally ill, probably for lack of information. The 'philosophical' suicide so beloved of the novelist, the poet and the pundit seems a rare occurrence.

Some 'physical' as opposed to 'mental' diseases have high suicide rates, but their individual contribution to the numbers of suicides is modest because they are uncommon in comparison with mood disorder and alcohol addiction. Their suicide rate is probably enhanced because of the effect of the disease upon mood rather than because of the disease itself. Some examples are given below.

Central nervous system disorders

These include:
    epilepsy (especially temporal lobe epilepsy), cerebral multiple sclerosis, head injury, Huntington's chorea, cerebral lupus, spinal cord injury, Parkinson's disease.

Gastrointestinal disorders

These include:
    ulcerative colitis, infective hepatitis, peptic ulcer.

Miscellaneous

These include:
    renal dialysis, limb amputation, laryngeal carcinoma treated by total laryngectomy.

End-stage cancer is often conjectured to be terminated by suicide, a fact not verified in the epidemiological literature.

Social

A high proportion of suicides live alone, or in non-private households or institutions; those living with others have strained relations and the happily married suicide is unusual. The incidence of 'life events' in the year preceding suicide is high and in the month before death about five times higher than in the healthy. A high proportion have recently moved house. An excessive number are unemployed, usually as the result of mental illness.

Medical

Nearly all suicides are in contact with their general practitioner; three-quarters have seen their doctor in the previous month, half in the previous week. A quarter are being treated by a psychiatrist. Poisoning by medically prescribed drugs is the cause of death in half the suicides in England and Wales.

Conclusion

There are two theories about the cause of suicide. The social theory states that suicide results from the disruption of the bonds which unite an individual with the society in which he lives. Disruption caused by the individual is 'egoistic' suicide, by society 'anomic' suicide. The mental illness theory states that suicide results when the illness induces suicidal action as a symptom, or as the considered way of ending dreadful, unbearable mental experience.

The social theory gains most support from the national statistics and the mental illness theory from clinical case studies. Mental illness appears to be necessary for a suicide to occur. Social influences probably work by adjusting a threshold for suicide in the mentally ill, but some social factors may influence the number of people who become ill.

Assessing Suicide Risk

Since no-one commits suicide without thinking of it, always ask about thoughts and plans for suicide – pills hoarded, a rope bought, the procedure lived through in imagination. What other preparations have been made – bills paid, wills made, insurance arranged, pets housed?

Depression, always present although not always severe, must be assessed.

Social influences are powerful. Living alone is a bad sign. So is a lodging or hotel. Look for one reasonably stable relationship as a prophylactic. The isolated person is the one to watch out for, even if living in a family setting.

Recent life events, especially those with a morbid significance, seem to enhance risk – death of a spouse for the lonely couple, loss of status for the ambitious, also events yet to come with a special unpleasant quality – appearing in court on a sex charge for a married man, impending marriage of a child for a lonely widow.

The epidemiological evidence can be used to adjust risk following the clinical assessment. A higher risk is attached to the male, the aged, the divorced and so on.

Illustrative Case Histories

Depression

Suicidal preoccupation is common in depressive illness; thoughts result in a suicide attempt and death only when they are intense or when meaningful personal relations are absent and when some loss or stress has recently occurred.

The patient came from a stable, Dublin, working class family, moved to England to work and led a happy life in an exclusive, childless marriage. Her first serious depressive illness began at the time of her husband's death when she was 54. Alone, she moved to the seaside and carried out the retirement she and her husband planned. Her symptoms were treated with barbiturates, and she took a fatal overdose of them on the anniversary of her husband's death.

Alcohol

Suicide in the alcoholic occurs after years of drunkenness have caused marital breakdown, decline in employment, money troubles and impaired health, both mental and physical. Depression is common, the suicide is rarely a surprise, being preceded by threats and attempts.

Alcoholism began in the 20's, death occurred at 47. The patient came from a heavy drinking professional family. After successful war service, he rose to the Higher Executive grade in the Civil Service, retiring because of alcoholism to a lower paid job two years before his death.

Epileptic fits, peripheral neuritis, gastritis, signs of dementia, a drunken driving conviction, battering his wife, quarrelling with his four children, and loss of status and income at work were the direct result of alcohol.

Depressed mood and frequent threats of suicide culminated in death from coal gas poisoning.

Schizophrenia

Suicide in schizophrenia occurs unexpectedly, sometimes at the instruction of hallucinated voices, sometimes to relieve unbearable alien mental experiences, sometimes because of depressed mood. Schizophrenics who kill themselves are young and have often had their established routine changed.

Schizophrenia developed at 21, death occurred at 38. The patient who was unmarried came from a stable working class family without history of mental illness, and had a good work record. Violence and crime, often at the command of voices, occurred in the early years, then he settled and spent ten years in a mental hospital. Four weeks before death he was moved to a seaside mental hospital near to his parents' retirement home. In the following month he moved wards twice and preparations were made for rehabilitation which had previously failed. Abusive voices and delusions of multiple marriage were signs of active illness but he was not depressed and had not spoken about suicide. He hanged himself in a public lavatory.

DELIBERATE SELF HARM

Attempted suicide and parasuicide are synonyms for non-fatal deliberate self harm (DSH), the preferred term because of its freedom from the aura surrounding the word suicide. Deliberate self harm has little to do with suicide.

Definition

There is no official definition for deliberate self harm in the Hospital Inpatient Enquiry which monitors admissions and discharges in England and Wales. In practice, intentional self damage can be inferred from the person's behaviour.

Epidemiology

The annual number of episodes of DSH is unknown. Reasonable estimates range from 100 000–150 000 hospital cases to 215 000 if the GP treated cases are included. Thousands more never reach medical attention. There are at least 25 times as many cases of DSH as of suicide. Deliberate self harm is the commonest cause for admission of a young person to a medical ward and therefore causes an enormous load on medical services. Similarly, the number of cases of DSH roughly equals new referrals of other conditions to psychiatric services.

Deliberate self harm by poison is a modern epidemic found in all western countries. Since 1961, the year attempted suicide ceased to be criminal in England, numbers have increased 5 to 10% annually, measured by discharges for poisoning (Fig. 8.3). Some levelling off occurred in 1977 and 1978. There is no association with the incidence of suicide, but there is an association with increase of prescriptions for psychotropic drugs. Free medicines have been proposed as the cause; but the rise of self poisoning occurred in countries without them.

The incidence of self poisoning has increased in both sexes and all age groups, excepting men over 65. Women of 15–24 years more than doubled their rate between 1968 and 1979 and they comprise a quarter of all admissions. Women account for 65% of admissions. The reasons are unknown.

The divorced have the highest rates of DSH followed by the married, single and widowed.

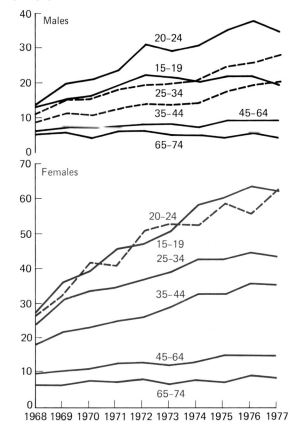

Discharge rate per
10,000 population

Fig. 8.3 *Age-specific hospital discharge rates for adverse reactions to medicinal agents in England and Wales; 1968–1977.*

Social class V has seven times the rate of deliberate self harm as social classes I and II.

In large cities DSH is associated with social disorganisation: mobility, overcrowding, eviction, violence, unemployment, crime and children in care.

Clinical

Self poisoning accounts for 90% of DSH and has become on that account virtually synonymous. Self laceration, hanging, shooting, drowning and the less common methods used in suicide itself comprise the remainder.

Analgesic, sedative, hypnotic and psychotropic drugs account for two-thirds of poisons used and most have been obtained with a prescription. Doses swallowed range from massive to trivial.

Barbiturates are less commonly used now, probably because of reduced prescription resulting from the profession's campaign against them. Antidepressants, in contrast, are more commonly used. About a third take alcohol as well. The proportion of patients admitted in coma has declined recently suggesting smaller overdoses or the increased use of the less toxic benzodiazepines or both.

Cases of DSH can, in theory, be divided into those who failed in their attempt to kill themselves and those who did it for other reasons – to go to sleep and ease the pain of an awful experience, to blackmail another person, to attract love and attention. And there are those who cannot say why and those who deny they did it.

In clinical practice the distinction is almost impossible. Perhaps 10% seriously want to die and another 10% wish in a less definite way that they had not survived. But the percentage of failed suicides, those who used dangerous methods, made preparations, left a note and so on, is only about 2%.

Mental illness is present in 10–20% of cases, almost all of it depression and anxiety. The 40% mentally ill reported in some studies is probably the result of including mental distress as mental illness. The remainder are not mentally ill. But about 15% are alcoholic and a high proportion have personality disorders, the proportion depending on the definition used.

The mental distress accompanying DSH is the result of quarrels with key people in about two-thirds of cases. The incidence of life events of a threatening and stressful nature in DSH is high and accelerates in the period immediately before the event. The self injury often seems an understandable response to a painful, distressing and sometimes hopeless predicament.

Outcome

One to two per cent of those who attempt suicide kill themselves each year compared with an expected value of about 0·005%. Ten to twenty per cent may eventually die of suicide. About a third of suicides have a history of an attempt.

Those 10–20% with mental illness have the prognosis for that illness.

Those with mental distress recover quite rapidly in a week or so from their acute symptoms and without treatment.

A repeat episode of deliberate self harm occurs in 15–20%. Some repeat many times. Repetition cannot be prevented by medical or social treatments.

Management

All patients should be interviewed to detect those with high suicidal intent or major mental illness. Such cases need urgent psychiatric referral. The rest may obtain relief by talking about their problems. If they want help, they can be directed to a social worker, a psychiatrist, a marriage guidance counsellor and so on.

Illustrative Case Histories

Failed suicide

A large overdose taken with evidence of planning to avoid detection, in the presence of serious depressive illness should be regarded as a failed suicide.

Depressive illness with conspicuous symptoms of abdominal discomfort and weight loss led, after 18 months of treatment in general practice, to referral to a consultant physician. After a negative investigation, an anxiety state was diagnosed and chlorpromazine prescribed. Two days later the patient, a married woman of 54, swallowed all the tablets she could find believing her husband would not return for 12 hours. She said, in hospital, that she wished she were dead. After four weeks of amitriptyline, normal health returned.

A serious overdose

An overdose can be taken to relieve, if only temporarily, the misery of domestic distress that has no apparent end to it. The hospital admission may, as in this case, result in effective treatment.

The patient, a woman of 34, previously divorced, was admitted after an overdose of 30 diazepam tablets. She took the tablets in front of her two small children after her boyfriend deserted her. These problems were identified: tension, insomnia, children out of control, family rejection, prosecution for theft, and debt. She smoked 40 cigarettes a day and drank 25 cups of tea to control symptoms.

Amitriptyline relieved her insomnia and improved her mood. Social work straightened out some problems. Five months after the overdose she was symptom-free and in control of her life.

A trivial overdose

An overdose can have as much psychiatric significance as throwing a plate at the wall. The medical significance can potentially be more serious.

An 18-year-old girl came home late smelling of alcohol. When her mother told her off she took 20 paracetamol tablets. Tears and guilt for all the trouble she caused were the conspicuous clinical signs in the hospital. A week later she was in normal health.

9

Alcoholism and Drug Dependence

ALCOHOLISM

Definition and Diagnosis

Descriptions of alcoholism indicate a variable syndrome. Presenting features may be physical, social or psychiatric in differing combination. The diagnosis of alcoholism is made when a person shows persistent, not necessarily permanent, harmful results from drinking ethanol. Essentially, an alcoholic is a person who goes on drinking when it is necessary to stop.

The diagnosis of alcoholism is therefore an appraisal of what has happened to the drinker; it is a statement of drink related phenomena. The diagnosis is not a recognition of a particular style of consumption (drinking pattern) or a pathological personality variant. Nevertheless, heavy alcohol consumption promotes a style of drinking which is different from that of moderate drinkers. Taking alcohol early in the day, drinking to relieve anxiety or tremor and a clockwork expectation of a continued supply are familiar marks of alcoholism. Lack of intoxication following a heavy dose of alcohol is a hall-mark. A random blood sample – for example, on presentation at a hospital casualty department – may settle the diagnosis. A blood alcohol of 150 mg/100 ml or higher without obvious physical effects – unsteadiness of gait and slurred speech – is strongly associated with pathological drinking.

There is no characteristic attitude or mental state which will identify a drinker as definitely alcoholic. However, drinkers who have harmful consequences from their habit often behave selfishly, minimise the quantity they take, or deny it altogether. Interest is narrowed so that drinking takes priority over other activities.

Events such as sexual rejection by a spouse are taken to be causes of increased alcohol intake, when they are really effects. It is common to hear that consumption only became troublesome on the departure of a wife; the woman will say that the drinking led to the parting. It is a truism that drinking leads to problems more often than problems lead to drinking.

The history given by the patient should be amplified by a third party account from a relative or friend – who may be sharply aware of what has happened during the period of heavy drinking. There is particular interest in the pattern of drinking – whether it is static or intermittent and whether there is an apparent relationship with psychological stress. The reported average quantity of alcohol consumed may not be accurate but it is worth asking what sort of drink is usual. Cheap sherry, cider and barley wine are taken for their alcohol content rather than their appeal to the palate. A family history of alcoholism may indicate genetic predisposition or a heavy-drinking subculture. Achievements and work record prior to the onset of faulty drinking may reveal traits of personality which will affect the choice of management.

The CAGE questionnaire is made up of four queries. Answering yes to two or more has been found to correlate with a diagnosis of alcoholism made after a traditional and more lengthy enquiry, providing that the patient's thinking or judgement is not altered by substantial psychiatric disorder, such as schizophrenia or brain damage.

1. Have you ever felt you should *cut down* on your drinking?
2. Have people *annoyed* you by criticising your drinking?
3. Have you ever felt bad or *guilty* about your drinking?
4. Have you ever had a drink first thing in the morning to steady your nerves or get rid of a hangover (*eye-opener*)?

Mental and Physical Examination

There is a wide variation in individual susceptibility to physical consequences; some, such as liver disease, may be sex-related. Tolerance – in the sense of diminished toxic effect as drinking continues – is almost universal. Withdrawal effects, such as morning tremor and anxiety, are much less constant.

Amnesic episodes are called 'alcoholic blackouts'. Failure of memory for a few hours – rarely for a day or more – happens during a drinking episode in which outward behaviour seems ordinary. During the episode, registration, i.e. awareness, is unaffected but retention – ability to recall what happened during the intoxicated state – is absent. Alcoholic blackouts are associated more with rapidly rising blood alcohol than an eventual high level.

Loss of tolerance – severe intoxication following moderate or small amounts of alcohol – is a late and inconstant phenomenon. Gastro-intestinal symptoms may indicate peptic ulcer, present or past hepatitis or pancreatitis – the last is often diagnosed relatively late.

Assessment of the mental state is directed first to the patient's attitude to his drinking, for this is central to treatment. How concerned is he? Is abstinence seen as threatening or potentially rewarding? Restlessness and a mood of anxiety or fear indicate a withdrawal state. A fatuous or dismissive attitude may be evidence of organic brain impairment or the result of years of detachment, due to intoxication, from the immediacy of ordinary experience. A test of present memory is vital, for patients with Korsakoff's syndrome often appear undamaged.

The physical appearance may also belie the underlying state. Obesity due to the high caloric value of ethanol may co-exist with a deficiency syndrome such as peripheral neuropathy. A tender hepatomegaly will indicate recent heavy consumption; signs of liver failure, a drinking history of many years; bruising may indicate falls while drunk, ill-treatment by others, or hepatic dysfunction.

Special investigations may reveal:

1. High random blood alcohol.
2. Macrocytosis without anaemia; not pathognomonic but useful because simply available.
3. Raised serum level of gamma-glutamyl transferase (GGT). This enzyme originates from the liver and is indicative of recent consumption; occasionally elevated due to other drugs. It has been used as a screening test in adolescents.
4. Electro-encephalogram (EEG) is normal unless brain damage is gross.
5. Computerised axial tomography (CAT) scan may show marked brain shrinkage in the absence of psychological evidence of intellectual impairment. The scan may slowly return to normal after up to a year of abstinence.

Pharmacology

Two organs are important in the breakdown of ethanol in the body: the liver because it is the only one which has an enzyme specific to its metabolism; the brain because it reveals disturbance of function most obviously. The similarity between the action of alcohol and general anaesthetics has suggested that the mechanism of its effect on the brain may be simply physico-chemical rather than a primary interference with neurotransmission. Brain function is depressed; there is no stimulant effect.

Figure 9.1 illustrates liver metabolism. Ethanol is converted to acetaldehyde by reaction with nicotinamide adenine dinucleotide (NAD), which is converted to the reduced state (NADH). This reaction is brought about by a specific enzyme, alcohol dehydrogenase (ADH). A separate dehydrogenase converts acetaldehyde to acetate, which is then metabolised in various sites, such as the liver, kidney and cardiac muscle. Two drugs, citrated calcium carbimide and disulfiram, stop the process midway by preventing the subsequent metabolism of acetaldehyde; this leads to a build-up of acetaldehyde, which causes unpleasant symptoms such as flushing, palpitations and nausea (the acetaldehyde reaction).

Causes of Alcoholism

There is evidence from studies of identical twins that genetic predisposition is a factor in the development of alcoholism. Equally, research has shown that the prevalence of alcohol related disorder in a community is related to average consumption. More interesting still is the observation that when the average level of drinking in a population rises, there is an excessive increase in the number of heavy drinkers. The inference is that susceptibility to alcoholism is graded but there may be a threshold level of consumption above which drink related problems are present in many individuals. Some individuals succumb even in a community of generally moderate drinkers. Others are recruited, probably disproportionately, as the general level of consumption is increased. The question of what level of drinking is acceptable for a particular group or community is complex (Fig. 9.2).

In wine producing countries, there is a sophisticated drinking pattern without prominent drunkenness. Alcoholics from such a background are often 'habitual-excessive' drinkers who show inability to abstain rather than 'loss of control' over their drinking. Manifest alcoholism is usually late

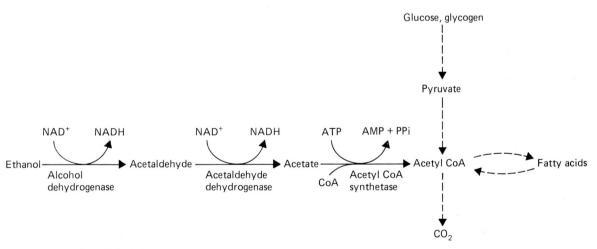

Fig. 9.1 *Metabolism of alcohol.*

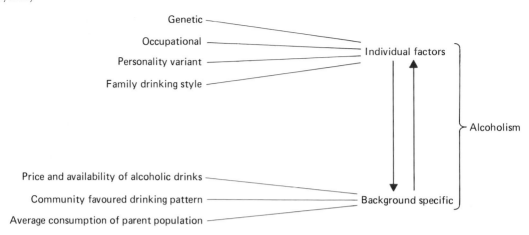

Fig. 9.2 *The alcoholic process.*

and characterised by physical disease, typically hepatic or neurological.

In many European countries, overall consumption is restricted by price and licensing laws. Alcoholism may then present as loss of control or binge drinking. Acutely disrupted behaviour is separated by periods of near abstinence.

Psychological dependence describes the use of alcohol to evade mental discomfort – such as feelings of anxiety or frustration. This may be the initial stimulus for some alcoholics but most develop a degree of mental reliance on the drug with time. Physical dependence is shown by the presence of withdrawal symptoms which respond to further alcohol; in contrast to psychological dependence, it is inclined to appear early in the drinking history or not at all.

Deaths from liver cirrhosis in different occupational groups are an acceptable comparative measure of incidence. Publicans have a mortality from liver cirrhosis which is almost eight times that of the general population; barmen have a rate which is twice the average. When alcohol is readily available at work, rates of alcoholism are increased. The difference between the publican and the barman in this respect indicates that availability is not quite the same as access. The

element of supervision experienced by the barman acts as an external control. Other groups with a raised incidence of alcohol problems include merchant seamen and members of the armed forces. In both these groups there is a tolerance, even approval, of heavy drinking combined with an absence of family restraint.

Complications of Alcoholism

A number of events may form distinct crises in the alcoholic process. Some are based strictly on organic change, others are cataclysms of personal adjustment. They are not all dose-related. The Wernicke-Korsakoff syndrome is rare; heavy drinking is common. Alcoholic liver disease is more common in women – perhaps related to a general tendency to autoimmune disorder.

Withdrawal phenomena

Usually these follow a halt to drinking and appear from twelve hours to a few days later. However, temporary lowering of blood alcohol, sometimes due to intermittent vomiting, can have the same result.

Alcoholic convulsions

These are grand mal fits which follow absolute or relative withdrawal from alcohol. They are not evidence of latent epilepsy; interval EEGs are normal. Treatment with anticonvulsants, such as phenytoin, can be tailed off a week or two after the fits have stopped.

Delirium tremens

This was first described in 1813 among spirit drinkers on the East Coast of England whose smuggled supplies were liable to interruption. Even with treatment, there is a definite mortality, from chest infection, hyperpyrexia or cardiovascular collapse. The onset, up to several days after drinking has stopped, is characterised by a mood of fearful anxiety accompanied by tremulousness, sweating and inability to sleep. Unchecked, this may develop into a restless delirium in which there is disorientation, visual hallucinosis, and thick speech whose content is hard to follow. The visual hallucinations are often of animals, reduced in size, perhaps behaving as humans. They sometimes entertain rather than frighten the patient. Signs of dehydration are present, as well as autonomic disturbance: thready pulse, pyrexia and sweating.

The cause of delirium tremens is probably a rebound over-arousal of brain activity. Alcohol has the effect of partial suppression of rapid eye movement (REM) sleep. When an habitual drinker stops his intake of ethanol, the REM pattern dominates sleep. The subsequent delirium could be thought of as vivid pathological dreaming which is complicated by biochemical disturbance. The latter is not well defined; dehydration and acute liver damage are often present. The EEG shows fast wave activity in contrast to other delirious states.

Treatment is symptomatic: fluid balance correction, prevention of fits and sedation. A number of drugs will control the delirium. Chlorpromazine is effective but must be accompanied by phenytoin to prevent fits. Chlordiazepoxide or chlormethiazole in reducing doses combine sedation with anticonvulsant action. Each of these drugs can produce dependence if prescription is continued unwisely and this is an especial danger with chlormethiazole. Water soluble vitamins (B and C) are given parenterally to prevent the added complication of the Wernicke-Korsakoff state.

Alcoholic hallucinosis

Auditory hallucinations without altered consciousness may occur while drinking continues. There is no relation to schizophrenia.

Wernicke-Korsakoff syndrome

This syndrome may be related to an inborn deficiency of transketolase activity which is only revealed in conditions of thiamine deficiency. See p.22 for clinical features.

Generalised brain damage

Although dilation of the ventricles and cortical atrophy are not uncommon in heavy drinkers, there is no evidence of an unselective, global dementia due specifically to alcohol. Tests of general intellectual ability show little change, although the development of a somewhat vacuous, shallow personality suggests frontal lobe damage. If such changes occur insidiously, then there is an explanation for the apparent disregard of risk and immunity to social pressure which is shown by some alcoholics at an earlier stage.

Depressive illness

Many alcoholics say they drink because they are depressed; the majority seem to be depressed because they drink. However, suicide is commoner in alcoholics than the general population, as is deliberate self harm (see Chapter 8).

It is likely that the social consequences of

alcoholism combine with biochemical effects to produce a pattern of depressive reaction which is mainly secondary to drinking and therefore not amenable to separate treatment.

Treatment of Alcoholism

The therapeutic attitude of those who wish to help individual alcoholics has to be straightforward, consistent and realistic. Attention is directed to methods of altering the drinking habit rather than rescue from the consequences. Most addicted drinkers are anxious and uncertain. Questions such as 'What do you fear will happen if you give up alcohol?' and 'What was it like when you tried to cut down?', will help to expose the reasons why drinking continues despite evident troubles.

Most authorities believe that an alcoholic drinking pattern is not easily converted to 'controlled drinking'; the aim of treatment would therefore be complete and permanent abstinence. In all cases, there needs to be an initial period of complete abstinence for six months. It is likely that ability to learn new behaviour is impaired during heavy drinking and this must cease to allow treatment a fair chance.

The setting in which treatment takes place is not critical, providing the therapist is informed. Out-patient counselling by a social worker can produce results equal to those obtained by treatment as an in-patient at a specialist alcoholism unit, providing there is reasonable family support. Self-help groups such as Alcoholics Anonymous can be effective, particularly where the illness is one of intermittent or bout drinking.

Detoxification, 'drying-out', as opposed to treatment in the longer term has a place in management, though repeated hospital admission for this purpose may be harmful. The alcoholic is encouraged to continue drinking in the mistaken belief that medical intervention will always restore health.

Prescribing psychotropic drugs, such as benzodiazepines, to take the place of alcohol has not been successful. Alcohol is generally added and the result is a mixed drug dependence with a considerable risk of harmful overdosage. A minority of patients may feel their resolve is strengthened, at least for a period, by taking citrated calcium carbimide which will evoke the acetaldehyde reaction if they drink. Eventually, a conscious, informed choice has to be made about future drinking.

Strength of Alcoholic drinks

A measure of spirits contains 10 g of absolute alcohol. The same quantity is contained in a half-pint of beer, and a drink of sherry or wine in an average sized glass (Fig. 9.3).

Various authorities have proposed 'safe' levels of drinking. These are higher for men than women because of women's liability to liver disease. The

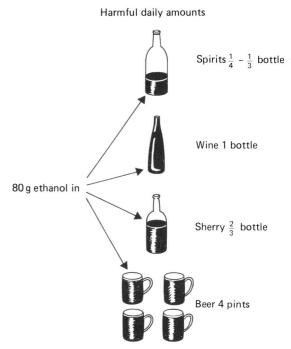

Harmful daily amounts

Spirits $\frac{1}{4}$ – $\frac{1}{3}$ bottle

Wine 1 bottle

80 g ethanol in

Sherry $\frac{2}{3}$ bottle

Beer 4 pints

Fig. 9.3 *Harmful daily amounts of alcohol.*

difficulty which is inherent to such estimates is that behavioural change following alcohol depends on such factors as speed of consumption and social context. Cirrhosis of the liver, though important, is not the only measure of harmful drinking. An estimate of a level of consumption which is almost always harmful is more to the point; 80 g or more of absolute alcohol daily is such a level.

DRUG DEPENDENCE

A large group of drugs have effects which lead to repeated usage. This includes substances such as nicotine which are harmful but permitted by law. The use of cannabis and lysergic acid diethylamide (LSD) is illegal and this increases desirability for people who feel out-of-step with their community. Adolescents who practise glue-sniffing emphasise this element of substance abuse. They discover that the strongest effect is to produce anxiety in adults who have no effective response to the habit. Amphetamines were used medically, as stimulants and antidepressives, until a tendency to produce paranoid psychoses was recognised. They are now used intermittently, without medical prescription, by individuals whose main dependence is to a sedative or narcotic drug. Cocaine is another central nervous stimulant which produces dependence. It is sensible to confine its use to local anaesthesia although it has been a constituent of analgesic mixtures for the terminally ill and may be prescribed legally by a doctor.

Opiate Dependence

Pharmacology

Morphine, diamorphine (heroin), pethidine and methadone have linked chemical structures and display cross-tolerance. That is, the withdrawal effects of one member of the class (in a dependent subject) are reduced by the other members. Each has numerous somatic effects. The mental effect is one of calm, slightly euphoric, mood, associated with a general freedom from discomfort and a flattening of emotional response. This is related to the attachment of morphine and its analogues to receptor sites which are normally available to endorphins.

Tolerance to this group of drugs is marked but it is lost within a few weeks of withdrawal. An addict who is unaware of this may take an accidental overdose.

The abstinence syndrome indicates physical dependence. Abdominal pain, vomiting and diarrhoea are accompanied by diffuse muscle cramps, increased secretion of mucus in the respiratory tract and watery eyes. The pupils dilate.

The speed with which such symptoms, or their prodromal signs, appear is the key to understanding physical dependency. A withdrawal reaction to heroin appears within six to eight hours. Reinforcement for an addict to repeat the drug is, therefore, prompt and strong.

In contrast, methadone has a slower rate of elimination. Unlike heroin, which crosses the blood–brain barrier rapidly, methadone is released into the circulation after it has accumulated in the tissues. The withdrawal reaction to methadone is correspondingly delayed for up to two days and is less severe. Morphine and pethidine occupy an intermediate place.

Treatment

The object is to enable the addict to live a contented life without drugs. A proportion of patients will not aim so high. A compromise objective may then be agreed, consisting of hospital admission, physical assessment, planned withdrawal of the primary addictive drug and substitution with oral methadone. A test for hepatitis B antigen is made before admission. Drug injectors have an increased risk of infective hepatitis and endocarditis.

During the withdrawal phase, oral methadone is given. Continued support and interest is needed following discharge so that the addict's way of life is diverted. If the plan is to continue prescription until a wish for a drug-free life is decided upon, methadone mixture (British National Formulary) is supplied. This provides a substitute which is not easily injected and, to some extent, reduces the mental effect induced by heroin.

Legal aspects

Medical practitioners are able to prescribe any drug, including heroin, to non-addicts. The Dangerous Drugs Act of 1967 limited the ability to prescribe heroin and cocaine for addicts to specially licensed doctors. Later acts oblige all doctors to notify the Chief Medical Officer of the Home Office when they believe, or suspect, that a person is addicted to certain controlled drugs – mainly opiates. This notification is what some patients refer to as being 'a registered addict'; it does not imply a statutory right to receive addictive drugs. It can be useful to know whether an individual is already notified and the Home Office will give this confidential information to a doctor.

10

Psychosomatic Medicine
With Special Reference to Eating Disorders

PSYCHOSOMATIC MEDICINE

The term 'psychosomatic' is not readily definable. This is in part because of historical changes in its application and in part because of its connection with philosophical problems of the 'mind–body' relationship.

From the 1930s to the 1960s the term was usually applied to some physical disorders which were held to be, to a significant degree, caused by emotional factors. These diseases, which included peptic ulcer, bronchial asthma, ulcerative colitis and essential hypertension, came to be called 'psychosomatic disorders'. As psychoanalysts were most enthusiastic in their study, so many conceptions of pathogenesis were couched in psychoanalytic theory. For example, it was suggested that a specific personality type or a specific psychodynamic conflict constituted the core (e.g. the wish to be independent versus the wish to be cared for) which, when impinged upon by a life situation directly activating this conflict (e.g. recruitment into the armed forces), led to the development of the disorder (e.g. peptic ulcer) in those who suffered a constitutional vulnerability of the organ in question.

These pioneering hypotheses proved difficult to study empirically but the scientific study of psychological factors in disease derived an important stimulus from them. Interest was engendered also by the observations of physiologists like Cannon on the visceral concomitants of emotion and the reports of Beaumont and H. G. Wolff on the effects of emotions on the gastric mucosa as observed in fistulous subjects.

More recently, questions have been posed which have proved more amenable to verification. These have included the following:

Do psychosocial factors such as major life events play a role in the onset of disease?

Are some of these factors more 'stressful' to some individuals than to others?

What psychological and physiological changes occur following exposure to stress? To what extent do they vary between individuals? To what enduring characteristics of the individual, both psychological and physical, are they related? To what extent are they subject to learning?

Can the changes above increase the vulnerability of the individual to the development of an illness? What intervening variables are involved?

Do psychosocial factors play a role in determining the outcome of established diseases?

The term 'psychosomatic' has emerged as one characterising an approach to illness rather than an adjectival description applied to certain disorders. This approach assumes that diseases have multiple causes and that there are often complex interactions between these causal factors and mediating processes.

The psychosomatic approach entails an examination of the relationships between biological, psychological and social variables as they pertain to disease – in aetiology, treatment and prevention.

'Mind–Body' Relationship

This fundamental issue needs to be addressed in a manner which allows progress to be made in a broader understanding of disease. A practical standpoint which may be adopted is one which recognises the terms 'physical' and 'psychological' as describing different 'languages' or sets of concepts which are based on different sets of observations. On the one hand somatic processes are described in 'physical language' (e.g. in terms of tissue pathology, biochemical changes) while on the other hand, psychological processes are described in 'psychological language' (e.g. in terms of cognition, mood, mental mechanisms). Many events can be studied by methods of both kinds, according to the aspect from which the events are viewed. An example is the phenomenon of 'arousal' (Fig. 10.1). It will be evident that 'arousal' cannot be understood as being simply 'physical' or 'psychological'.

The 'psychosomatic approach' accepts that there is an interplay and sequence of processes pertaining to disease, some of which are best viewed psychologically, others physically and others from both aspects. The view which is allowed to predominate for any particular phenomenon is that which is most adequate in its explanatory value. Prominence may change as new observations are made and new hypotheses tested. Often the two views prove complementary. It also follows that in theory any disease may be subject to both viewpoints.

This approach will underly the discussion of obesity and anorexia nervosa below.

OBESITY

There is no precise criterion of obesity. In general terms it is a condition caused by an excess amount of adipose tissue. A number of indices are used to describe its severity but the commonest is observed weight as a percentage of desired weight.

Mortality rates tend to rise in proportion to the degree of overweight. For example, the Framingham study, a prospective epidemiological investigation of the development of cardiovascular disease, showed such a relationship. Most of the risk appeared to be exercised through an association with obesity of hypertension, hyperlipidaemia and impaired glucose tolerance.

Causation

The short-term regulation of hunger and satiety and the long-term control of weight are extremely complex. Many influences on these functions have been identified, ranging from the level of sociocultural factors to CNS neurotransmitter activity.

In some societies where poverty and disease are endemic, obesity is a valued characteristic. In

Physical Language	Phenomenon of 'Arousal'	Psychological Language
Changes in blood pressure, heart rate, muscle tension.		Changes in level of alertness
Changes in skin conductance.		Changes in intensity of motivation.
Changes in reticular activating system.		Changes in efficiency of task performance, e.g. visual discrimination.
Desynchronisation of the EEG record.		Sensitive to amount and variety of sensory input, sleep deprivation, etc.

Fig. 10.1 *The description of 'arousal'.*

industrialised societies there is a relationship between socioeconomic status and the prevalence of obesity. It is more common in lower status groups and less common in higher status groups.

General population studies of obese individuals have failed to show an increase in psychoneurotic characteristics compared with normal weight subjects, at least in the middle aged, 20–50% above standard weight. In fact they tend on some measures to score less than normals, supporting the popular notion of 'jolly fat'. The clinic obese, however, usually weighing much more, show a high level of psychological disturbance.

At the psychological level a hypothesis has been proposed which links obesity with a greater than normal sensitivity to environmental food cues and a diminished sensitivity to inner physiological cues to hunger and satiety. This 'externality' theory has however been challenged. An alternative view has been presented which holds that obese people are more likely to be restricting their food intake to lose weight ('dietary restraint') and that it is this restraint which accounts for much of 'obese behaviour'. Restraint, it is argued, is exercised in the face of a 'set point' for weight mediated via the hypothalamus which in the obese person is high. The restraining obese person may thus be 'statistically overweight' but 'biologically underweight'. External food cues, anxiety or alcohol may serve to overcome restraint and in fact lead to overconsumption of food under these conditions.

At the biological level, numerous influences on weight control have been identified. There is, for instance, evidence to support a role in hunger and satiety for food palatability, 'glucostatic' mechanisms (dependent on the rate of cellular uptake of glucose), 'lipostatic' mechanisms (dependent on the body's state of fat stores, possibly mediated by blood fatty acids and prostaglandins), and 'thermostatic' mechanisms (dependent on changes in body heat). These controls are ultimately mediated through the CNS. Anatomical destruction of the ventromedial hypothalamus (VMH) in experimental animals produces hyperphagia and obesity whilst destruction of the lateral hypothalamus (LH) produces hypophagia and wasting.

A number of abnormal eating states, differing from each other in subtle ways, can be produced by more circumscribed lesions affecting particular neural pathways (e.g. medial forebrain bundle, nigrostriatal tract). These findings and the results of the administration of specific neurotoxins (e.g. 6-hydroxydopamine) or of direct application of neurotransmitter agents to brain areas have suggested that certain neurotransmitters are involved in the regulation of hunger and satiety. High CNS controls also operate since lesions of limbic lobe structures (e.g. amygdaloid complex, hippocampus) as well as of the neocortex may produce marked changes in eating behaviour. In man the operation of genetic factors in weight determination is shown by a familial tendency to obesity, the evidence from twin studies and also from adoption studies, where a closer weight correlation has been reported between adoptees and their biological parents than with their adoptive parents.

Interest has focused recently on the role of adipose tissue in obesity. There is histological evidence that the adipose tissue of some obese persons, particularly those whose obesity began in early life, may contain more fat cells than does the adipose tissue of non-obese persons or of persons whose obesity began during adult life. This may be the explanation for the observations that childhood obesity, in which fat cell hyperplasia is more likely, persists so strongly into adult life. This would be because the achievement through dieting of a reduction in less enlarged fat cells to a subnormal size is much more difficult than a reduction of more enlarged cells to a normal size. Fat cell hyperplasia may be irreversible and thus constitute a sort of 'biological trap' for obesity. This hypothesis has been challenged but if it is correct then there are important implications for prevention.

Clinical Aspects

A useful classification of obesity is the following:

1. Lifelong, childhood onset type: constitutional factors are probably important and sustained weight loss is difficult to achieve.
2. Later onset type: psychological and social influences are probably more important, e.g. decline in physical activity.
3. Obesity associated with endocrine or metabolic disease, e.g. hypothyroidism, Cushing's syndrome, Froelich's syndrome.
4. Obesity associated with rare diseases of the hypothalamus interfering with regulatory centres.

Patients presenting clinically with severe obesity frequently show high levels of psychological disturbance. Affective features are common as are intense feelings of self disgust. Interpersonal relationships and sexual activity tend to be restricted and it sometimes appears that the obesity serves to conceal problems in these areas, since these may emerge in distressing forms after weight loss. Depression is a recognised complication of weight reduction in some patients. A disturbance of body image is often apparent where, even after weight loss, patients see themselves as bigger than they really are.

There is marked variation of eating behaviour between patients. Often there is a stereotyped pattern for a particular individual, e.g. insomnia and hyperphagia at night with morning anorexia. Emotional and personality factors may play an obvious role, particularly when the patient is exposed to stressful life situations.

Treatment

Assessment

The patient's motivation for weight loss requires careful assessment. Not infrequently, weight loss may be seen unrealistically as the solution to all of life's problems.

A detailed weight history needs to be obtained including a description of the associated eating patterns, the results of previous attempts at weight loss and psychological concomitants of these.

Treatment approaches

1. The simplest way of ensuring weight loss is by in-patient supervision. With a low calorie diet (600–800 kcal) a reduction of 8–10 kg in 40 days can be expected. However, in the absence of intensive follow-up care, weight tends to be regained.
2. The most effective approach on an out-patient basis is a behavioural treatment regime aimed primarily at altering the patient's eating pattern. Significant weight loss can be achieved (e.g. 10–15 kg over one year) although in most cases weight tends to be regained later.

   Behavioural measures might include:

   a) The patient monitors his behaviour by keeping a detailed diary of what he eats and when and where.
   b) Eating is confined to specific locations and times.
   c) A full place is set at the table whenever or whatever he eats.
   d) Eating is made a 'pure experience' by separating it from all other activities, e.g. reading, watching television.
   e) The 'topography' of eating is altered, e.g. slowing down, frequent pauses.
   f) The salience of eating cues is diminished, e.g. by keeping food out of sight.

Exercise is a useful adjunct. In addition to increasing energy expenditure, it may also decrease appetite in the obese and increase the metabolic rate.

Enlisting the help of a co-operative spouse or family member may also prove valuable.

3. Although appetite suppressant drugs often facilitate short-term weight loss, particularly if combined with dietary advice, long-term benefit is unusual. Dexamphetamine and phenmetrazine may induce dependence, whereas fenfluramine and diethylproprion, equally effective, do not. Some studies have shown intermittent therapy with diethylproprion (four weeks on, four weeks off) to be as effective as continuous treatment. Fenfluramine is not suited to intermittent administration since depression is common following withdrawal.

4. Self-help groups: Overall, success in the long-term is limited and drop out rates are high.

5. Surgery: Bypass surgery may be justified for some of the extremely obese. Physical complications can be serious, but psychosocial benefits to patients are considerable.

Outcome: Overall, the long-term outcome of treatment is disappointing but there is significant individual variation. Unfortunately, there are no helpful predictors of outcome.

ANOREXIA NERVOSA

Anorexia nervosa is an illness mainly affecting young girls after puberty and is characterised by:

1. Severe self induced weight loss.
2. Amenorrhoea.
3. A specific psychopathology in which the principal feature is a morbid fear of fatness and pursuit of thinness.

The disorder is not as rare as was believed in the past. The incidence of new cases referred to psychiatric services alone was found to be 1·6 per 100 000 population per year for N.E. Scotland in 1969. There is also some evidence that the incidence is increasing although this is at least in part due to better recognition of the disorder in recent years. A recent study of London schoolgirls aged 16–18 years revealed a prevalence of 1 in 250.

Causation

The influence of sociocultural factors is reflected in the probably increasing incidence of the disorder, the scarcity of reports in coloured populations and in a social class bias favouring its appearance in social classes I, II and III. The idealisation of a thin body shape in the West and the consequent preoccupation with dieting may act as a trigger in predisposed girls who, after commencing to diet, find they are unable to stop. That a concern with body shape may be an important predisposing factor to the development of the illness is supported by the high prevalences found in ballet schools (up to 6%) and modelling schools. Clinically the patient's behaviour appears to be generated by her desire for thinness and abhorrence of fatness. Bruch has drawn attention to some important psychological characteristics of patients with anorexia nervosa. These include a pervasive sense of personal ineffectiveness and inability to influence one's fate, and an apparent loss of normal sensitivities to internal bodily and psychological cues to hunger, satiety and the appreciation of body shape. In the face of her deep sense of lack of autonomy the patient strives to exercise control and finds that she can do this most successfully in the sphere of dietary restraint, being aided in this by her insensitivity to internal regulating cues.

There is experimental evidence to suggest that patients with anorexia nervosa are more likely than normal controls to overestimate the size of their body dimensions.

The disorder may also be understood in broader psychological terms as a retreat, both biological and psychological, from the challenges presented by puberty. These include demands for greater independence and for dealing with emergent sexuality. A girl, psychologically unprepared to confront these changes, may discover that self-starvation and emaciation constitute a defensive mechanism which ensures the preservation of a child-like, simple existence in which these challenges can be avoided. For example, in addition to the cessation of menstruation and the flattening out of feminine curves, a decline in sexual drive is experienced, from which the girl may acquire considerable relief.

Family factors may also play a role. A delicate family homeostasis may have been reached whose continuing viability depends on the maintenance of the 'status quo'. A child's emergence through adolescence to independence may threaten this balance and result in the appearance of distressing conflicts. A starved, child-like girl may guard against this development.

Some psychological disturbances may be a product of the malnutrition. It is, for instance, a common observation that mood often improves considerably with weight gain under treatment. Hypothalamic function has been intensively studied since this is intimately involved in the regulation of eating, sexual function and temperature, all of which are abnormal in anorexia nervosa. Although many disturbances of hypothalamic function can be demonstrated (e.g. changes in sex hormones, growth hormone, adrenocorticosteroids, etc.) it is difficult to determine whether these are primary aspects of the disorder or secondary consequences of the malnutrition. With weight restoration, demonstrable abnormalities of growth hormone secretion, of hypothalamic–pituitary–adrenal function and of temperature regulation generally revert to normal.

The strongest evidence for a primary hypothalamic disorder lies in the disturbance of the hypothalamic–pituitary–gonadal axis. In many cases there is a dissociation between this and weight in that amenorrhoea may precede substantial weight loss, while menstruation may not resume for months or even years after the patient has regained a healthy weight. Patients with anorexia nervosa show a failure of release of the gonadotrophins, LH and FSH, from the pituitary and have low circulating oestrogen levels. Luteinising hormone (LH) and follicle-stimulating hormone (FSH) release in response to intravenous luteinising hormone releasing hormone (LHRH) is impaired. The evidence suggests that the primary defect is at the hypothalamic level since more prolonged LHRH infusion will result in a normal response indicating intact pituitary function. As the patient regains weight, sex hormone function is generally recovered in a definite sequence. There is a gradual increase in the levels of FSH and LH and the response of these gonadotrophins to administered LHRH is restored at about 75% of standard body weight. Next, a return of the negative feedback response of LH to oestrogens can be demonstrated. Finally, a positive feedback to oestrogens is re-established which results in the mid-cycle surge of LH associated with ovulation. This final stage of recovery may be long delayed after the patient's weight has been restored to normal and this appears to be related to persistent psychopathology. Figure 10.2 illustrates some of the possible causal factors in anorexia nervosa.

Clinical Features

The illness usually begins in a girl aged 14 to 18 years but the onset may be earlier or later, even up to the menopause. Anorexia nervosa also occurs in males in a ratio of about 1:15 females. The following features are of special importance.

Weight loss

This may be very rapid, e.g. 20 kg in three to six months. Weight reduction usually begins with dieting. Soon, however, it progresses beyond reasonable bounds. Carbohydrate containing

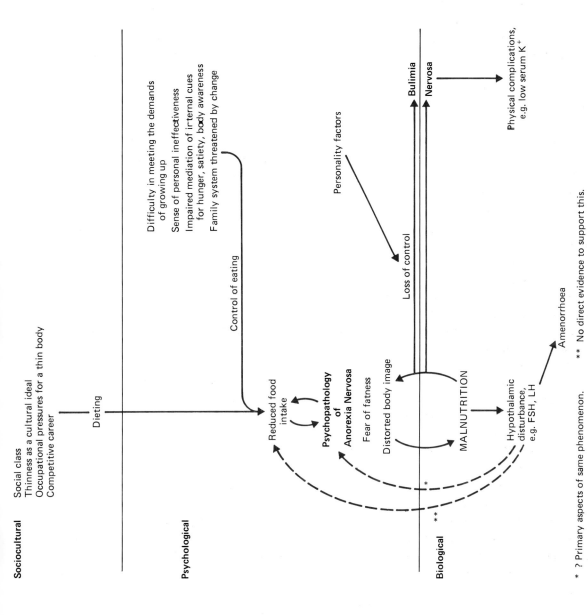

Sociocultural   Social class
                     Thinness as a cultural ideal
                     Occupational pressures for a thin body
                     Competitive career

Dieting

Control of eating

Difficulty in meeting the demands
of growing up
Sense of personal ineffectiveness
Impaired mediation of internal cues
for hunger, satiety, body awareness
Family system threatened by change

Psychological

Reduced food
intake

**Psychopathology
of
Anorexia Nervosa**

Fear of fatness

Distorted body image

Personality factors

Loss of control

**Bulimia
Nervosa**

Physical complications,
e.g. low serum K⁺

MALNUTRITION

Hypothalamic
disturbance,
e.g. FSH, LH

Amenorrhoea

Biological

*

**

* ? Primary aspects of same phenomenon.   ** No direct evidence to support this.

Fig. 10.2 *Some factors in the causation of anorexia nervosa.*

foods are specially avoided and the patient's meagre intake may be largely composed of vegetables, cottage cheese and black coffee. She may resort to subterfuges aimed at avoiding meals or to the disposal of food. Self-induced vomiting, purgative abuse and excessive exercise may further accelerate weight loss.

Amenorrhoea

This usually follows substantial weight loss but it may precede it. Loss of periods is usually received with indifference by the patient. In the male amenorrhoea is replaced by diminished sexual interest and potency.

Psychopathology

The central theme is the patient's morbid fear of becoming fat. A fear of losing control over eating is usually expressed and the pursuit of thinness may entail the establishment of a margin of safety in case 'over-eating' should occur. A maximum weight can be elicited from the patient above which she will not countenance going and which is very low in relation to her healthy weight. Particular sensitivity may be revealed about certain body parts, e.g. hips, thighs. A disturbance of body image may be betrayed by her belief, in the face of emaciation, that she is of normal weight or even fat. She minimises the extent of her food avoidance. Anxiety or guilt associated with eating is often expressed while preoccupation with thoughts of food and weight may be extreme. Figure 10.3 illustrates, in a drawing, a patient's feelings about her body size.

Other features are evident. Profound changes in personality are usual. The patient's life becomes more constricted socially and she may become more reclusive at home. Sexual contact is avoided. Family relationships become strained as attempts to coax, bully or bribe her to eat meet with failure. Schoolwork may be attacked with fierce determination and long hours of study. Depressive,

anxious and obsessional symptoms may be prominent. Obvious physical hardships resulting from the malnutrition tend to be denied or minimised. The girl eventually consults a doctor only reluctantly and after persistent entreaties from relatives and friends.

Physical examination discloses signs of severe emaciation with the disappearance of subcutaneous fat and with bony prominences thrown into sharp relief. The hands and feet may be cold and blue even in a warm room. Hypothermia, hypotension and bradycardia are noted. There is excessive growth of dry downy hair (lanugo)

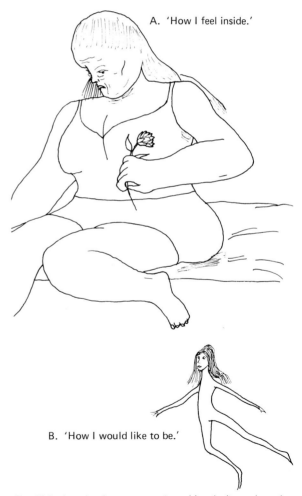

A. 'How I feel inside.'

B. 'How I would like to be.'

Fig. 10.3 *A patient's representation of her feelings about her body, drawn when she weighed 40 kg.*

particularly over the nape of the neck, forearms and legs.

The diagnosis is usually straightforward on clinical grounds.

Hypopituitarism is not associated with marked wasting.

'Bulimia Nervosa'

This is a variant of anorexia nervosa and often represents a chronic phase of the illness. The main features are:

1. Irresistable urges to overeat, usually huge quantities of previously 'forbidden' foods.
2. Compensation for overeating with self-induced vomiting and abuse of purgatives.
3. The same psychopathology – a morbid fear of fatness.

Gorging and vomiting may occur many times a day. Between these episodes the patient usually starves herself. Patients in this phase of the illness may have a relatively normal weight and may also menstruate. A more outgoing personality, often with less impulse control (evident in self-mutilation, alcohol abuse, shoplifting), is more often noted in these patients than in those with 'typical' anorexia nervosa. Depression and feelings of self disgust may be very prominent.

Serious physical complications may arise from habitual vomiting and purgation. Particularly dangerous are electrolyte disturbances including hypokalaemia. Tetany, epileptic seizures, urinary infections, renal failure and intermittent salivary gland swelling may also occur.

Treatment

There is no specific treatment for anorexia nervosa but general measures achieve at least short-term correction of the malnutrition and save life.

The most important initial aim is to secure enough co-operation from the patient to allow treatment to commence. This may be difficult when illness is denied by the patient but a skilled and understanding physician can usually achieve this, perhaps after a few interviews.

Out-patient treatment alone is unlikely to succeed unless the patient is genuinely motivated and family support can be enlisted. Admission to hospital is usually necessary for the short-term goal of weight restoration. A compulsory order is rarely required for this.

In hospital, nursing treatment is crucial and requires careful planning. Skilled nurses can establish a relationship of trust with the patient based on an understanding of her experiences. This relationship is combined with supervision of all meals and the prevention of attempts to dispose of food. After a week or so the patient can be persuaded to eat meals containing 3000 kcal or more per day and she will gain 1–2 kg per week. Psychological support is required from the medical team throughout. As weight gain occurs, supervision and restrictions are relaxed. There is little place for drug treatments. On occasions, small doses of chlorpromazine may be useful for a particularly agitated patient. Skilled nursing has rendered tube feeding obsolete.

By the time of discharge, usually after 6 to 12 weeks in-patient care, the patient will have achieved a healthy weight and may show considerable improvement in mood and attitudes to her weight. A year or more of out-patient supportive psychotherapy will usually be necessary. The aims are to help the patient to tolerate normal weight and to explore and change some of the psychological and social difficulties associated with the illness. The support and involvement of the family may prove extremely important.

The treatment of bulimia nervosa is less well established. Intractable self-induced vomiting may require admission to hospital. Long-term supportive psychotherapy aimed at helping the patient to accept a healthy weight and to establish a

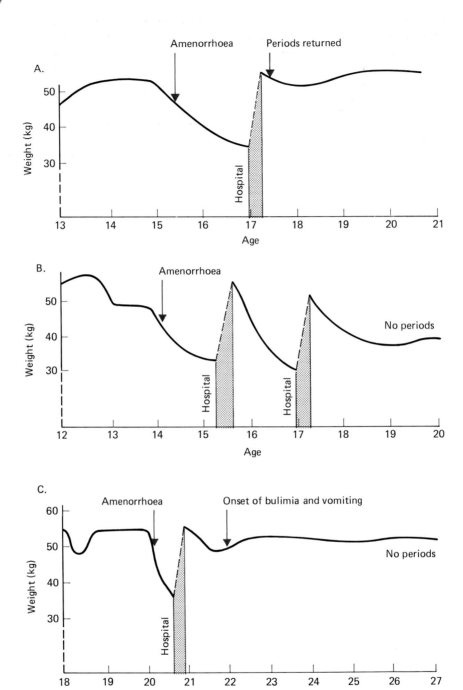

Fig. 10.4 *Weight histories of three patients illustrating the variety of outcome in anorexia nervosa.*

regular pattern of food intake is usually necessary. If it is successful, craving for food and bulimia will be reduced. Behaviour therapies may prove useful as may the involvement of family and friends.

Outcome

The illness often lasts 2–4 years. The mortality rate is about 5% with suicide probably now the commonest cause of death. The short-term prognosis for weight gain with treatment is excellent. The long-term prognosis is more difficult to gauge.

In a follow up of severely ill patients, at least four years after in-patient treatment, 40% were found to be recovered, 27% had a low body weight or menstrual irregularity and 29% suffered from a very low weight and amenorrhoea. Seventy to eighty per cent recovery is expected for less ill patients suitable for out-patient treatment alone. A poorer prognosis is associated with a later age of onset, a longer period of illness, a poor premorbid adjustment and the presence of bulimia and vomiting. Figure 10.4 shows some common outcomes of the disorder.

11

Psychosexual Disorders

SEXUAL DYSFUNCTION

The term sexual dysfunction is used to describe any persistent impairment of sexual interest or response.

Normal Sexual Interest and Response

Three stages of normal sexual response have been identified (Fig. 11.1). During sexual arousal a number of physiological changes occur; these are described below.

Vascular changes produce erection in the male, and genital engorgement, clitoral enlargement and lubrication in the female.

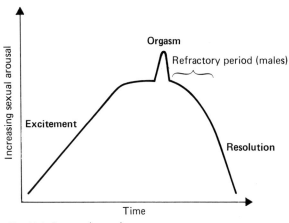

Fig. 11.1 *Stages of sexual response.*

Neuromuscular changes include elevation of the testes in the male, retraction of the clitoris in the female. Orgasm includes physical events and subjective sensations. There are two phases of orgasm in the male. Seminal and prostatic fluid enters the urethral bulb (emission), and then is ejected from the urethra in a series of spurts (ejaculation). In the female, similar muscle contractions occur. During resolution the physiological changes of arousal are gradually reversed. In the male this stage includes a refractory period of variable length (from 15 to 30 minutes at 15, to 24 hours or more at 80) before sexual arousal can recommence. There is no corresponding physiological refractory period in females, and some women experience a series of orgasms in close succession.

Adequate androgen levels are essential for the full development of sexual function in men. However, withdrawal of androgens in adulthood (e.g. through castration) may not cause erectile impotence, although the ability to ejaculate may be lost. In females, androgens maintain sexual drive, and oestrogens facilitate normal genital responses to sexual stimulation.

Types of Sexual Dysfunction

Primary sexual dysfunction is present from the onset of sexual activity, secondary dysfunction occurs after a period of adequate sexual function. A dysfunction may be situational in that it occurs in one setting (e.g. with a partner) and not in another (e.g. during masturbation).

Most forms of sexual dysfunction can be categorised according to the phase of sexual interest or response which is affected (Table 11.1).

Impaired libido

Disorders of sexual interest are far more common among women than men, at least in terms of patients who seek medical help. Men more often complain of problems concerning sexual performance. Impaired libido is often associated with disorder of sexual response. For example, a man who lacks interest in sex may also have difficulty in obtaining an erection. However, some patients with impaired libido can respond normally.

Erectile impotence

Failure of erection may be partial, when incomplete erection occurs or when full erection occurs but is lost when intercourse is attempted. When the dysfunction results from psychological factors, the man usually reports that erections occur on waking in the morning or when he is having sexual thoughts, and the onset of the disorder is likely to have been fairly sudden. Erectile impotence occurs more often in middle aged and older males.

Premature ejaculation

If a man regularly ejaculates before vaginal penetration this is clearly premature. Otherwise the term is best reserved for cases where the man feels he has little or no control over when he ejaculates. It typically occurs in younger men and is probably due to psychological factors.

Ejaculatory failure

This is relatively uncommon. Sometimes the dysfunction occurs only with a partner, ejaculation being possible in solitary masturbation. In other cases ejaculation is impossible under any circumstances (except perhaps sleep). Sometimes the complaint is of slowness in ejaculating. Ejaculatory failure may also be caused by drugs, particularly antihypertensives and monoamine oxidase inhibitors (see below).

Female impaired arousal

Disturbance in the excitement phase of sexual

Table 11.1

Types of Sexual Dysfunction in Men and Women

Phase of sexual response	Sexual dysfunction	
	Men	Women
Interest or desire	Impaired libido	Impaired libido
Excitement	Erectile impotence	Impaired arousal
Orgasm	Premature ejaculation Retarded ejaculation Pain on ejaculation	Orgasmic dysfunction
Other	—	Vaginismus Dyspareunia

response in women is characterised by impairment of genital swelling and lubrication during sexual activity. Although this is very likely to occur in association with impaired libido, as a distinct clinical syndrome it is usually the result of physiological factors such as oestrogen deficiency. It typically occurs following the menopause when there may be marked atrophic vaginitis.

Orgasmic dysfunction

Failure to achieve orgasm may range from total failure to mild situational anorgasmia. In the latter condition women reach orgasm only with very prolonged stimulation. The extent of orgasmic difficulty which is seen as constituting a problem varies considerably from woman to woman, and is influenced by contemporary attitudes towards female sexuality. Certainly many (if not most) women do not always achieve orgasm but are content with their sexual responsiveness.

Vaginismus

This is inability to have sexual intercourse, or difficulty in doing so, because whenever vaginal penetration is attempted spasm of the pubococcygeal muscles surrounding the vaginal introitus occurs. Most women with vaginismus have a simple phobia concerning penetration, but are otherwise responsive; in other cases the symptom is part of a much wider sexual problem.

Dyspareunia

Pain during sexual intercourse may be the result of lack of vaginal lubrication; in this case the pain is usually experienced at the vaginal introitus and often disappears as intercourse proceeds. However, pain may occur because of organic pathology, such as a poorly repaired episiotomy, vaginal infection or endometriosis. Pain on deep penetration is highly suggestive of an organic cause. Often such pain persists after sexual intercourse.

Causes of Sexual Dysfunction

Sexual dysfunction can result from many causes. They may be classified into psychological and physical causes. In many cases with a physical cause, psychological factors are also relevant. Causal factors can also be sub-divided into:

(i) remote or distant factors in an individual's background which have made that person vulnerable to developing a sexual problem in adulthood.

(ii) precipitants, following the occurrence of which the sexual dysfunction has appeared; and

(iii) maintaining factors which serve to perpetuate the problem, of which anxiety is the most important (Fig. 11.2). Sometimes there has been no obvious precipitant.

The contribution of physical factors to sexual dysfunction is being increasingly recognised. For example, erectile impotence occurs in a third to a half of men with diabetes, usually as a result of neuropathy affecting the autonomic nerves which mediate erectile function. It can be the presenting symptom of diabetes. Some women with diabetes may experience orgasmic dysfunction. The neurological pathways which mediate sexual response may also be interrupted by disorders which afflict the spinal cord (e.g. multiple sclerosis, trauma). Patients with ileostomies or colostomies may have sexual difficulties because of the embarrassment which results; rectal surgery may result in damage to the sacral nerves involved in sexual response. Sexual problems may follow myocardial infarction, often because of an expectation that a heart attack automatically ends sexual activity. Angina during sexual activity may be another factor. Sexual problems are also common after mastectomy, usually because of the woman's sense of unattractiveness.

Many drugs interfere with sexual interest and response (Table 11.2). Some affect erectile function because of their anticholinergic effects (e.g. tricyclic antidepressants), others interfere with sympathetic mechanisms (e.g. beta-blocking

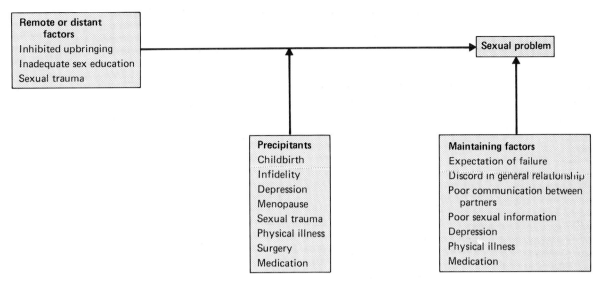

Fig. 11.2 *Some causes of sexual dysfunction.*

antihypertensives), while in some cases the mechanism is unclear (e.g. bendrofluazide). Alcohol abuse can profoundly affect sexual function by causing neuropathy, hypogonadism or depression. Sexual dysfunction is also often associated with drug abuse.

Management of Sexual Dysfunction

Before instigating any form of treatment an adequate assessment must be carried out.

Assessment

When assessing a couple, it is usual to interview the partners separately. This encourages each partner to reveal important information which might not be disclosed in the presence of the other partner. The first aim is to obtain a clear idea of the nature of the presenting problem. Thus, a woman may complain of lack of orgasm during intercourse, only for it to emerge that her partner ejaculates immediately after penetration. Questions should be asked about the patient's sexual development, including the attitudes of the family to sexuality, where information about sex was gained and the extent of the patient's knowledge, the nature of previous sexual relationships and any problems which were encountered, masturbation, including attitudes towards it, and homosexual interest or experience. A history of any medical and psychiatric disorders should be obtained, and any recent or current drug treatments noted. The patient should be asked about the use of alcohol and illicit drugs. A careful check should be made for any current psychiatric disorder, such as depression or alcoholism. The couple's general relationship must be thoroughly assessed to determine whether the sexual problem is the result of general disharmony.

A physical examination may be indicated, especially in a women presenting with vaginismus or dyspareunia, or a man with erectile impotence or ejaculatory failure. Physical investigations may be necessary, including fasting blood sugar (in erectile impotence), and blood tests for testosterone and gonadotrophin concentrations (luteinising hormone and follicle-stimulating hormone) if hypogonadism is suspected. An abnormal testosterone

Table 11.2

Drugs which may Cause Sexual Dysfunction

Anticholinergics		Propantheline
Antidepressants	Tricyclics	Amitriptyline
	Mono-amine oxidase inhibitors	Phenelzine
Antihypertensives	Ganglion blocking	Guanethidine
	β-blocking	Propranolol
	Central-acting	Methyl-dopa
Anti-inflammatory		Indomethacin
Diuretics	Thiazides	Bendrofluazide
Hormones	Oral contraceptives	
	Steroids	
Hypnotics	Barbiturates	Sodium amylobarbitone
Major tranquillisers	Phenothiazines	Thioridazine
Minor tranquillisers	Benzodiazepines	Diazepam

result is an indication for obtaining a serum prolactin level to rule out hyperprolactinaemia.

Treatment

Sexual dysfunction is amenable to treatment when the problem is not the result of major disturbance in the couple's relationship, when there is no serious psychiatric disorder (including alcoholism or drug abuse), and where there is sufficient motivation. Patients with sexual dysfunction secondary to physical illness can often be helped considerably by counselling.

For some patients only brief counselling will be necessary. This includes those whose problems are the result of inadequate information. The doctor can then help with advice and information.

For other patients more intensive treatment, or sex therapy, will be indicated. The approach used will depend on whether there is a partner willing to be involved in treatment. In 1970 Masters and Johnson, working in the USA, introduced an approach to sex therapy which is now used widely in the UK, often in a modified form. After careful separate assessments, the partners are seen together. Treatment may be carried out by one therapist, or by male and female co-therapists. The couple are presented with a simple formulation of their problem, including an explanation of its probable causes. They are asked to avoid intercourse temporarily and given instructions in carressing exercises to carry out at home. The couple begin with general carressing excluding the genitals, and then involve the genital areas during the following weeks. The couple are instructed in special methods to deal with certain sorts of dysfunction. An example is the stop–start technique of premature ejaculation, in which penile stimulation by the female partner is intermittently maintained according to the level of the male's sexual arousal. The partners are advised how to improve their communication, both in general and during sexual activity. When progress has been made the couple are then instructed on how to resume sexual intercourse, including an intermediate stage where penile insertion occurs but there is no movement.

Sex therapists need specialist training. Sex therapy is not just a series of exercises. Couples usually need counselling to help them recognise and modify obstructive attitudes or beliefs. They often need education, because ignorance and misinformation contribute to sexual difficulties.

A good outcome is obtained with approximately two-thirds of couples taken on for treatment. Vaginismus and premature ejaculation respond well. Poor prognosis is often associated with disharmony in the general relationship, and psychiatric disorder in one or other partner.

Help can also be provided for the individual with sexual dysfunction who does not have a co-operative partner. Women unable to achieve orgasm, and men with premature ejaculation or ejaculatory failure, can be helped with instructions about masturbation, and by counselling about sexuality. It is difficult to help a man with erectile impotence who does not have a partner.

Hormonal treatments are of limited use in the treatment of sexual dysfunction. Testosterone administration to men with erectile impotence is only effective if there is marked impairment of testicular function. Treatment with bromocriptine can be effective where erectile impotence is the result of severe hyperprolactinaemia. Other drug therapies are not very effective, except where used to treat an underlying disorder (e.g. depression).

Patients with sexual dysfunction associated with physical disability, and their partners, can receive considerable help from counselling. Where the dysfunction is permanent, a couple can learn to adjust and continue to have a rewarding sexual relationship. Patients anxious about the implications of a physical illness (e.g. ischaemic heart disease) for their sexual functioning can similarly be helped.

SEXUAL VARIATIONS

The term sexual variation is applied to any sexual activity that is preferred to, or displaces, hetero-sexual intercourse, or one that involves very unusual methods of arousal. A wide range of sexual variations exist. They are regarded as deviant when they violate the norms of society. Few sexual activities receive universal disapproval (this includes incest), whereas many others, such as homosexuality or transvestism, only evoke strong protest where the age of consent is contravened or one partner is unwillingly involved. The medical profession tends to be involved in the treatment of sexual variations where these are regarded as being the consequence of illness. The position of doctors in this respect can change with time, as has happened in recent years with homosexuality.

Homosexuality

Homosexuality is not an all-or-none phenomenon. Some individuals are entirely homosexual in orientation and only have homosexual relationships, others may be attracted to their own sex but rarely get involved in homosexual relationships, and some people appear to be bisexual, showing similar interest in homosexual and heterosexual relationships. Distinction can be made between homosexual acts, which include any feelings or activity of an erotic nature directed towards a person of the same sex, and homosexual identity, which involves acceptance of such erotic feelings or activity as an integral part of one's personality.

The prevalence of homosexuality in the general population is uncertain. Some 40 years ago in the USA, Kinsey found that 7% of men aged 30 were largely or entirely homosexual. It has been estimated that between 2 and 4% of the female population are homosexual.

Until the Sexual Offences Act of 1967, all forms of male homosexuality were illegal in this country. Under the Act the legal age of consent for male homosexuality is 21. Homosexual behaviour between consenting males in private is not illegal provided both men are aged 21 or more. There are no laws specifically concerning female homosexuality, except in the armed forces.

Why homosexuality occurs is unknown. It has been suggested that genetic factors may make an individual susceptible to becoming homosexual if he or she is exposed to certain environmental influences. Abnormalities in exposure of the male brain to androgens, either pre- or post-natally or both, could also lead to vulnerability to other factors. No reliable differences have been found between homosexuals and heterosexuals in their hormonal make-up or physique. Disturbed relationships with parents have also been implicated in the aetiology of homosexuality, with little supporting evidence. In addition, anxieties about heterosexuality and the conditioning of homosexual fantasies through masturbation may play a role in the development of homosexual interest.

Female homosexuals rarely seek help from doctors and male homosexuals seek medical help less often than in the past. There are several reasons why help is still sought. First, adolescents who are developing homosexual interest may seek help because of the concern about this either on their part or that of their parents. Second, some men try to escape from their homosexual interest through marriage but later discover that this is not a satisfactory solution. The third and probably the most frequent reason for seeking medical advice is difficulty in accepting homosexual inclinations. Development of heterosexual orientation is more likely if the man has had any past heterosexual interest, does not regard his homosexual interest as an integral part of his personality, is relatively young, and is highly motivated. The use of aversion therapy has not proved very effective. In addition, such approaches raise ethical and moral issues. Fourthly, homosexual men can develop sexual dysfunction just as can heterosexual men. Finally, homosexual men are at increased risk of developing venereal disease (especially syphilis) and hepatitis B infection.

Other Sexual Variations

Exhibitionism is behaviour in which gratification is sought through genital display to members of the opposite sex, usually strangers. Indecent exposure is the term used to describe the legal offence. It is the most common sexual offence in this country, and frequently involves young males. Two types have been described. The first includes inhibited young males who fight the impulse to expose themselves, find it irresistible, expose a flaccid penis, gain little pleasure from the act and feel guilty afterwards. The second includes individuals who are less inhibited and often of sociopathic personality. They expose in a state of excitement, masturbating an erect penis, and enjoy the act with little subsequent shame or guilt. Their behaviour often contains a sadistic element. They are likely to show other psychiatric and sexual disturbances. The reaction of the victim is important to the exhibitionist, who would prefer her to show shock or curiosity; lack of interest tends to diminish his satisfaction. Some exhibitionists take considerable risks, especially when they have current difficulties in their life. Indeed, some exhibitionists welcome being caught. Usually the individual's sexual adjustment is poor and sexual dysfunction is often found in either the man or his partner.

Fetishism refers to sexual behaviour in which an object, usually a particular form of clothing, is the primary source of sexual arousal. It is almost confined to males, and is closely related to transvestism, or cross-dressing. The transvestite gets pleasure and usually sexual satisfaction from wearing female clothing. A transsexual is an individual who has a powerful urge to change sex. There is a major disturbance in the person's gender identity (his or her sense of being a male or female), which is often apparent from an early age and which is very resistant to change. Transsexuals may be of either sex, although male transsexuals are more common. Transsexuals usually seek surgery and hormonal treatment to bring about sex re-assignment.

Paedophilia refers to sexual activity in which one or both partners is under the legal age of consent. Some individuals are specifically attracted to sexual activity with young and immature partners. The behaviour may be confined to either heterosexual or homosexual activity, but some paedophilia occurs between family members. Actual violence is rare.

Incest, or sexual activity between family members, is probably far more common than would be thought from the frequency with which cases come to the notice of the police. Sibling and father–daughter relationships are the most frequent forms of incest. Many factors may contribute to the development of a father–daughter incestuous relationship, including personality disorder and alcoholism in the father, parental disharmony, and collusion by the mother.

Management of Patients with Sexual Variations

Before offering treatment it is most important to be clear, first, what the patient wants, and second, what is feasible. For example, there is usually little point in trying to modify well-established homosexual interest in a middle aged man who has had no previous interest in heterosexual relations. A thorough history should be obtained along the lines described for patients with sexual dysfunction. Apart from clearly identifying the nature of the sexual variation, evidence of any sexual dysfunction which might be sustaining the individual's interest in the sexual variation should be sought.

In many cases the best approach is to help the patient improve his general sexual adjustment, with little attention paid to the sexual variation, especially if he has a partner who is willing to co-operate in treatment. The approach described for management of sexual dysfunction can then be employed.

Where the patient seeks direct help with his sexual variation, a variety of means of improving self-control and reducing interest in the behaviour may be considered. Aversion therapy, in which small electric shocks to the patient's arm are paired with deviant sexual fantasies, is rarely used, although good results have been obtained in the treatment of fetishists and transvestites. Covert sensitisation, in which aversive images are paired with deviant fantasies, is another approach. The patient might be taught to practice in imagination other things he might do when the variant sexual desire occurs. Some patients, such as exhibitionists, have been helped by meeting regularly in a group to discuss their difficulties and means of overcoming them. Patients whose sexual variations seem to be in part the result of inadequate social skills which prevent them establishing a normal relationship with the opposite sex may benefit from social skills training. Finally, libido-suppressing drugs, of which cyproterone acetate is the most useful, occasionally may be indicated, particularly for the patient who fears his behaviour will bring him in conflict with the law but does not mind the general impairment of libido which is likely to occur.

Some patients will not wish to give up their behaviour but may seek help in adjusting to the problems it brings. Such patients can often be best managed by suggesting they contact one of the organisations specifically established for people with their particular interest.

12

Psychological Methods of Treatment

Patients presenting with psychological problems account for many consultations in general practice. Psychotropic drugs are over-prescribed for such patients, often because of a feeling of impotence on the part of the doctor who has no experience in psychological methods of treatment. This chapter is an introduction to the principles involved in these important treatment methods.

Psychological treatment can be broadly divided into behavioural and psychodynamic. Behavioural treatment concentrates on overt behaviour, attitudes, feelings and thoughts which are assumed to have arisen from faulty learning. Psychotherapy is more concerned with the meaning of symptoms, which are assumed to arise from conflicts between persons or within a person. These two approaches to treatment have much in common. Both stress the importance of the relationship between therapist and patient, and require the patient's active involvement.

Insight-orientated psychodynamic individual or group therapy and complex behavioural treatment usually require referral to specialist psychiatric services. Behavioural treatments have tended in the past to be the province of psychologists. Dynamic therapies were carried out by doctors or trained analysts. The need for psychological treatments can never be met by highly trained and expensive psychiatrists and psychologists. The use of other professions, nurses, social workers and others is therefore a necessity. With adequate, but

often short periods of training, these groups have been shown to be effective in conducting psychological treatments. Medical students should acquire a general knowledge of the principles of treatment and the skills to carry out supportive therapy, counselling (e.g. marital counselling) and simple behavioural therapy.

Family and marital therapy are not covered in the text but many of the principles described for other therapies are applicable.

BEHAVIOURAL PSYCHOTHERAPY

Behaviour therapy has its roots in experimental psychology and learning theory, although in practice therapeutic methods are based almost entirely on the principle of reinforcement.

Principle of reinforcement

In Pavlov's classical conditioning experiment a bell was sounded whenever food was presented to a dog. The response of salivation became conditioned to the sound of the bell. At about the same time, Watson in America demonstrated that fear of animals could be conditioned in a small child and May Jones showed that simple phobias (e.g. fear of spiders) in children could be reduced by repeated association of the feared object and a pleasurable experience (e.g. eating a sweet). These ideas had little clinical impact until Wolpe developed the concept of reciprocal inhibition, in which one response (e.g. relaxation) inhibits another response (e.g. anxiety). He devised 'systematic desensitisation', which is a treatment of phobic anxiety combining a step-by-step approach to the feared object or situation with the use of relaxation to inhibit anxiety.

Operant conditioning was shown by Skinner to be a process in which spontaneous behaviour produced by an animal or person is rewarded (e.g. by food or praise) and therefore increases in frequency. A behaviour which is punished decreases in frequency.

In practice, it is assumed that any pattern of behaviour which persists is being reinforced and no attempt is made to fit behaviour patterns into operant or classical conditioning models. Reinforcement may be from within the patient (e.g. frightening thoughts about death increasing anxiety) or result from the response of others (e.g. praising a child for desired behaviour). The patient's behaviour may be reinforcing, an example being the phobic patient who runs away from the feared situation. The consequent decrease in anxiety reinforces the fear of the situation. Here reduction of anxiety acts as a reward.

An everyday example of reinforcement occurs when little John sees some sweets at the supermarket checkout. He starts asking his mother for sweets, she refuses, he shouts, she refuses, he throws himself on the floor and screams. Mother gives in, and buys him some sweets. If this sequence of behaviour is often repeated, little John learns that screaming produces things that have previously been refused.

Behavioural analysis

Before a treatment programme (Fig. 12.1) is begun, the therapist must decide what the problem is and whether behaviour therapy is appropriate. A programme of treatment is devised and discussed with the patient. The patient's and close relative's

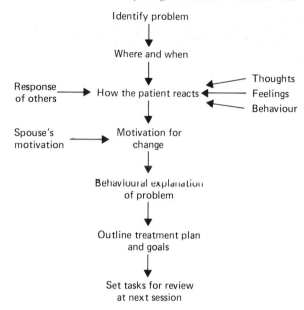

Fig. 12.1 *Behavioural treatment plan (initial session).*

motivation for change must be assessed, as any treatment programme will require their active co-operation.

A patient with agoraphobia will be used to illustrate behavioural analysis and treatment. The first step in the analysis is to ascertain the circumstances in which anxiety occurs. In agoraphobia this would be away from home, especially in crowds or buses.

A list of circumstances is drawn up, ranging from the least to the most anxiety-provoking. Then the therapist looks at the patient's reaction to each circumstance with reference to: (i) physical symptoms like palpitations or sweating, (ii) frightening thoughts, such as 'I am going to faint', 'If I collapse nobody will know who I am or where I live', (iii) the patient's response, which might be to panic and leave a crowded shop, and (iv) how others respond, e.g. the husband does all the shopping, encouraging his wife to stay at home to avoid distress.

The patient and spouse (or other key person) must be motivated for change. Where the husband of an agoraphobic woman prefers his wife to remain at home because he has developed a life-style which excludes her, he is likely to undermine the treatment programme. The woman, after years of staying at home, may have adapted to this way of life, and rewards for change will need to be explored. Rewards might be visiting friends or taking up old social interests such as dancing. Motivation is important as behaviour therapy relies heavily on the patient practising what has been learnt in the treatment sessions. This homework is the most important component of treatment in agoraphobia.

Once a clear picture of a patient's problem is elicited, the problem is discussed with the patient as simply as possible. The way in which the problem started and what the patient and others do to make it continue are explained. The treatment programme and its rationale are outlined and some preliminary tasks are set which can be reviewed at the next session. In this type of treatment the therapist's role is often that of a teacher helping the patient to understand the problems and to learn new ways of thinking and behaving to master the problems.

Behavioural treatment

In agoraphobia the treatment programme might consist of teaching the patient some of the following strategies:

  (i) relaxation to reduce anxiety by inhibiting it,
 (ii) remaining in an anxiety-provoking situation so that the anxiety has time to reach a peak and then fade,
(iii) reassuring self-talk, for instance, 'My heart is racing because of anxiety, I am not having a heart attack',
 (iv) distracting herself from anxiety by engaging in another activity, like looking into a shop window and thinking about what she sees.

All these strategies encourage patients to feel in control of their symptoms. In agoraphobia the most important component of treatment is repeated exposure to feared situations. This exposure needs to be for one to three hours a day, usually in a graded fashion, sometimes more rapidly, depending on the patient.

The two main components of behavioural treatment are anxiety reduction and learning new behaviours. The latter needs to be extended further in many patients, with advice about altering a life-style previously restricted by illness, and here the involvement of the patient's family may be crucial.

Uses of behavioural psychotherapy

Behavioural treatment has been shown to be effective in obsessive-compulsive neurosis, anxiety states, phobic anxiety states, sexual dysfunction and for nocturnal enuresis and phobias in children. It is also used in social skills deficits, marital therapy, alcoholism, social rehabilitation in chronic disorders such as schizophrenia and mental handicap, compulsive gambling and other disorders of impulse control, but in these disorders its effectiveness is less certain.

It is important to emphasise that a knowledge of behavioural principles is valuable in understanding patients in many different situations. It is not just a body of techniques to be applied to patients with certain disorders.

DYNAMIC INDIVIDUAL PSYCHOTHERAPY

The important features of dynamic psychotherapy are the therapeutic nature of the patient–therapist relationship and the search for meaning in the patient's symptoms.

Present day psychotherapy has its basis in psychoanalysis, an intensive treatment involving 50-minute sessions, four or five times a week. The patient's problems are explored through free association in which the patient says whatever enters his mind. The therapist's main involvement is in interpretation of transference (the patient's relationship with the therapist), in order to produce insight (understanding). Psychoanalysis is a time consuming and unproven treatment not generally available in the health service.

Individual psychotherapy is now heavily influenced by social learning theory and humanistic-existential ideas. Sessions are usually once weekly and therapy may be long term (over one year) or focused on a particular problem over a contracted number of sessions.

Uses and aims

Patients selected for individual therapy may have problems in their relationships with others, have low self-esteem, feel unfulfilled, be troubled by non-adaptive character traits (such as lack of assertiveness) and suffer from a range of neurotic symptoms. They must be motivated for therapy and be able to think in psychological terms. A patient who believes his mood swings are entirely due to disturbed biochemistry is unlikely to benefit from dynamic therapy.

The aim of therapy is to increase self-understanding, leading to symptom relief and changes in problems such as those outlined above. Many therapists now discuss specific goals for problem changes with the patient so that progress can be reviewed within therapy.

Therapeutic strategies

The patient–therapist relationship is the most important component of treatment. The therapist should be himself without revealing his own personal life. He needs to be aware of how the patient is reacting non-verbally, the meaning behind what the patient says, and how he is feeling towards the patient and the patient towards him. He needs to be continually looking at the process behind the content, at what is

happening between the patient and therapist, rather than what is being said. An example might be the patient repeatedly bringing up a violent film he had seen when he is really angry with the therapist.

Within the patient–therapist relationship 'transference' will develop. Transference is a psychoanalytic term that describes the way in which the patient relates to the therapist as a result of his relationships with important people in his remote or recent past. For example, a patient might try to appease the therapist because his own father was an invalid and he was always afraid of making him ill. This childhood experience might have led to a self-effacing attitude to authority. By being able to understand this link and become assertive with the therapist the patient could alter his relationship to authority figures.

The analysis of defences is another component of therapy. Defence mechanisms (Fig. 12.2) are the means by which the ego, the executive component of our personality, protects itself from internal or external threats. These mechanisms are unconscious, and largely adaptive in protecting us from uncomfortable emotions. However, they can be maladaptive if they hinder a person's normal functioning. An example is excessive denial leading to repeatedly avoiding difficulties in a marriage.

Looking at the patient's defences leads to the uncovering of hidden feelings that are denied because of the distress which they cause by

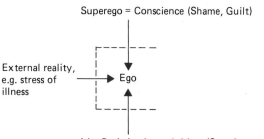

Fig. 12.2 *Defence mechanisms.*

becoming conscious. The feelings might be of anger or sexuality towards a close person.

Transference, defence mechanisms and hidden feelings are brought into the patient's understanding by interpretation by the therapist. Other strategies the therapist may employ are clarification, linking and confrontation. Clarification is to elucidate what is being said and what the patient is trying to convey. Links are made between the patient's behaviour in the session and outside, between feelings towards the therapist and other people, between present and past difficulties. The patient is confronted with his acting-out behaviour such as coming late for sessions because he is angry with his therapist.

Although emphasis has been laid on various strategies, the therapeutic nature of the patient–therapist relationship remains paramount. To promote this relationship the therapist must be caring without being possessive. He must promote trust, a feeling of security and confidentiality in which the patient is able to be honest and open in a way which is not possible in ordinary family or social interaction. Finally, the patient must be helped to become independent of the therapist. This is achieved by the patient forming a framework of understanding of his personality which he can use himself without the therapist's help.

GROUP PSYCHOTHERAPY

Man is a social animal spending much of his time in groups. An awareness of the importance of interpersonal factors (relations between people) as well as intrapersonal factors (a person's relation to his inner world) in psychological problems has led to the increasing use of group therapy in psychiatric practice.

As well as a wide variety of long-term group psychotherapies (between one and two years), groups are used with in-patients, in self-help (Alcoholics Anonymous), in teaching skills (e.g.

social skills), in increasing self-awareness (e.g. encounter groups), and in a wide variety of other settings.

Described here is a long-term group therapy based on the principles of interpersonal learning and derived from a model used by I. D. Yalom. Much that is described is applicable to other long-term groups and also to groups in general.

Uses and aims

These are similar to those of individual psychotherapy. However, the patient must be able to accept treatment in a group and some patients are unsuitable because of severe withdrawal or shyness.

Preparation for a group

There is good evidence that patients who are prepared for a group with explanatory hand-outs and discussion are less likely to drop out of treatment. Patients are told that there will be six to eight people in the group including the therapist, that meetings will be once a week for an hour and a half, and continue for about 18 months. New members may be added if anybody leaves the group. Members are expected to attend regularly, to be honest and open, to respect confidentiality and not to socialise with other members outside the group. This promotes group security and cohesiveness. Patients are led to expect that the first three months will be difficult.

In addition, many patients are aided in using the group by setting goals for themselves. These might be increasing assertiveness, becoming independent of parents, or becoming more at ease with one's homosexual orientation.

The group develops

The therapist is active in establishing a 'here-and-now' focus. This focus is on what is happening in the group to members rather than what is happening outside the group, 'out there', or in relation to the patient's past, 'back then'. 'There' and 'then' will be appropriate at times but too much time spent on crises in the person's outside life or on archaeological exploration of his past is unhelpful. The patient will learn about himself by recognising how he behaves and feels in the group, getting feedback from others and trying out new ways of behaving. For example, Brian is constantly interrupting, not listening, talking about himself. His reason for coming into the group is that he cannot make friends. Other members point out that he is irritating them by ignoring their needs. He starts to listen, to take an interest in others. Other members notice this, and start to express warmth towards him. This process would probably take many months.

As in individual therapy the emphasis is on process, i.e. what is happening between people, rather than content, i.e. what is being said. The therapist will repeatedly point out the process and as the group progresses other group members will pick up this skill.

Groups go through certain stages (Fig. 12.3) before reaching the stage of maturity in which most therapeutic work is done. These stages are returned to intermittently throughout the group especially at times of stress, e.g. when new members are introduced. There is a stage of dependence on the therapist, deriving from his healing status and the lack of structure in the group. As he is revealed as a fallible human being who does not have all the answers he is criticised by the group members. This may help patients who suffer from an unreasonable fear of persons in authority. At this time the group is often a place of conflict and competitiveness as members strive for dominance, with arguments about who is and who is not getting enough of the group time. The final stage involves intimacy where patients test whether the group will accept their personal feelings and thoughts. Acceptance increases trust and a feeling of closeness, enabling the patient to be more self-disclosing.

Therapeutic factors

These factors have been distilled from clinical opinion and research into what seems to be important in therapy.

Group cohesion decreases drop-outs and makes patients feel they have benefited. A cohesive group gives the patient a feeling of being accepted and cared for, and enables the patient to take risks. Patients learn how their behaviour is perceived by others in the group. Feedback encourages insight and the group supports the individual's attempts to change.

Initially, advice-giving is a prominent feature of the group but lessens as relationships in the group become less superficial. Patients derive support from a feeling of 'being in the same boat'. This universality may be important to those who have felt their problems as unique. There is learning by identification by seeing how other people tackle their problems or express feelings. Here the therapist may act as an important model for emotional expression. Catharsis, the release of emotion, is now seen as having little value unless followed by intellectual understanding. As with individual therapy, transference both towards the therapist and other members may occur. The opportunity to help others gives confidence. This may be especially useful for those people who view themselves as in constant receipt of help from others. This active involvement in the treatment of others is also beneficial in that seeing others improve gives hope for one's own change.

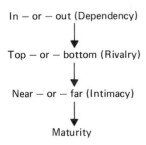

Fig. 12.3 *Stages in group therapy.*

Many of these factors are applicable to less intensive group therapies. For instance, universality, identification and hope might be particularly emphasised in self-help groups.

SUPPORTIVE PSYCHOTHERAPY

All the dynamic psychotherapies emphasise the therapeutic nature of the doctor–patient relationship. However, whereas most psychotherapies are aimed at fundamental change in the patient's relationship with himself and others, supportive therapy is aimed at maintaining the status quo. It is the most frequently used psychological treatment in general practice, in psychiatry and in the care of patients who have chronic social, physical or psychological problems. The aim is to help the patient to cope with problems, to remain independent and to use help appropriately.

Uses and aims

Psychiatric patients may be chronically handicapped by neurosis (e.g. chronic anxiety, depression with somatic complaints), by functional illness (e.g. schizophrenia), or by enduring personality traits (e.g. obsessional). Such patients are always vulnerable to stress and have little capacity for major change. Here supportive psychotherapy can help the patient function as well as possible, prevent relapses, increase self-esteem and help him set himself realistic goals.

Components of therapy

Supportive psychotherapy is not just common-sense advice and reassurance. Little has been written on this type of therapy but certain strategies are important.

(i) The patient can be reassured by explanation of symptoms. For instance, knowing about palpitations might reduce panic induced by fears of dying from a heart attack.

(ii) The patient may need guidance about ways of tackling practical issues such as claiming financial benefits.

(iii) It may be useful to help the patient make appropriate use of help. This often involves teaching the patient to communicate needs directly rather than indirectly through behaviour such as self-poisoning.

(iv) Self-esteem can be increased by looking at past achievements, and by paying special attention to anything the patient does well at present.

(v) Patients should not be encouraged to aim for more than they are capable of.

(vi) Emotional expression is usually encouraged but must be accompanied by discussion to aid understanding. For instance, it may help a man's tension symptoms if he is able to recognise his anger with his employer.

The patient should be encouraged to use other supports such as social clubs, self-help groups or day-care attendance. The therapist should also involve the family, the most immediate source of help for most people.

Danger of dependency

What is healthy dependency? Patients with chronic disabilities do need to depend to a certain extent on other people. However, over-dependency on one person can be destructive. When a therapist leaves, the over-dependent patient feels unsupported and goes into crisis. A patient may make increasing demands which cannot be met by one person so that the therapist feels exhausted and withdraws. Over-dependency can also increase passivity in the patient so he becomes less able to cope.

Dependency can be reduced by making sure that other supports such as the family are actively encouraged. Over-authoritarian advice-giving should be avoided. Many therapists can be seduced by the feeling that only they understand the patient and convey this feeling to the patient. This is unlikely to happen if the therapist is in regular discussion with others involved.

Setting up supportive psychotherapy

The essence of supportive psychotherapy is regular sessions. These may be only 15 minutes a month, but the regularity helps the patient contain problems between sessions. The limits of therapy must be carefully outlined including the discussion of criteria for extra sessions or use of the telephone in emergencies.

Preparation of a problem list (Fig. 12.4) in discussion with the patient helps to structure therapy. This list should contain a wide variety of psychological, physical and social problems, and each problem can be reviewed regularly to assess progress.

Intervention in crisis

The principles outlined here are applicable to all patients in crisis. Any person, however capable, will be unable to cope if under severe stress. Crisis intervention aims to help the patient cope with a problem in a mature and adaptive way. It is assumed that if an adaptive solution is found then this will lead to better problem-solving in the future.

An example of a crisis is the death of a supportive friend for a woman with chronic marital problems. Initially, the therapist would provide support by listening and allowing emotional expression. A knowledge of the normal process of bereavement would help the therapist to give the patient understanding of her feelings. Help is given with practical steps to find other supports. The goal would be an effective adaptation to the loss, rather than maladaptive behaviours such as overdosing with drugs or alcohol abuse.

Problem	Action
1. Chronic anxiety symptoms.	1. Explain symptoms. Encourage acceptance of symptoms. Teach relaxation techniques.
2. Intermittent abuse of prescribed medication.	2. Prescribe minor tranquillisers for short periods only (prescribing only by general practitioner).
3. Lack of support (non-involvement of husband).	3. Attempt to involve husband. Arrange day centre contact once a week. Involve volunteer visitor. Monthly out-patient contact.
4. Eldest child unhappy at school.	4. Encourage patient to see school-teacher, school counsellor.

Fig. 12.4 *Illustrative problem list.*

RESEARCH INTO PSYCHOTHERAPY

In behaviour therapy, with its roots in experimental psychology, there is much research activity. An emphasis on well-defined problems and goals for treatment has made controlled experimental design much easier than in dynamic psychotherapy. Comparison of behavioural treatment with dynamic psychotherapy has demonstrated that it is a more effective therapy in some well-defined conditions, e.g. phobic states, obsessional disorders. However, in only 10% of psychiatric patients requiring psychological treatment is behaviour therapy the treatment of choice. In behaviour therapy it has been possible by altering treatment variables in a controlled way to determine what are the important factors in treatment. For instance, in agoraphobia repeated exposure to feared situations has been shown to be more important than other factors in treatment.

It has long been debated whether the dynamic psychotherapies produce speedier and greater improvement than would be expected by 'spontaneous recovery'. Is improvement in therapy just due to changes in the person's external circumstances during treatment? The weight of evidence now suggests that psychotherapy is beneficial. However, it is less certain which type of psychotherapy is suitable for which patient. Outcome is difficult to measure as dynamic psychotherapy aims at more than relief or control of symptoms. The advent of short-term and goal-orientated therapies makes it easier to assess outcome, even if goals are defined in psychoanalytic terms.

13

Pharmacological and Other Physical Treatments

Drugs contribute greatly to the relief of suffering caused by mental illness, but they are rarely the complete answer to a patient's problem. They should be regarded as important aids to overall management.

Classification of Psychotropic Drugs

A psychotropic drug is one that influences mood and other psychological functions. Some years ago the World Health Organisation proposed a simple classification with five categories of drug (Fig. 13.1).

A single drug may be classified in more than one category and some drugs, such as lithium, do not fit comfortably into any category. Only drugs from the first three categories are considered in this chapter.

I Neuroleptics (antipsychotic drugs)
II Anxiolytic Sedatives (predominantly benzodiazepines)
III Antidepressants (tricyclics, newer compounds, MAOIs)
IV Psychostimulants (amphetamines) ⎫ Not in general therapeutic use
V Psychodysleptics (LSD, cannabis, etc.) ⎭

Fig. 13.1 *Classification of psychotropic drugs.*

Overprescribing of Psychotropic Drugs

There is a great deal of concern over the excessive prescribing of psychotropic drugs, in particular anxiolytic sedatives and antidepressants. Many factors contribute to this, but it is the doctor who prescribes and, especially in the case of the family doctor, some of the difficulties he faces help determine overprescribing. These include insufficient time, lack of training in psychotherapeutic methods and the demands of patients who see drugs as the panacea for all their problems. The consequences of overprescribing include more unwanted effects, a greater number of cases of self-poisoning (including accidental poisoning in children) and increased cost to the health service.

UNWANTED EFFECTS OF PSYCHOTROPIC DRUGS

The price paid for progress in drug treatment is a large number of unwanted effects. There are interactions between the drug and the patient's psychological and pathophysiological state, but they may also be influenced by psychological and social factors. Unwanted effects occur in normal therapeutic dosage and may be classified as shown in Table 13.1. Toxic effects also occur from drug interactions, drug administration by the wrong route and overdosage.

Table 13.1

Types of Unwanted Effects

Type	Example
An excessive degree of a wanted effect	Over-sedation due to an antianxiety drug
An unavoidable part of the pharmacological spectrum	Anticholinergic effects of a tricyclic antidepressant
A hypersensitivity or allergic reaction, mediated through antigen–antibody mechanisms	Exanthematous rash caused by a phenothiazine
An idiosyncratic reaction occurring in those genetically or constitutionally predisposed	Convulsions induced by an antidepressant

Predisposing Factors

These include age, with the very young and the very old being particularly vulnerable, and pre-existing physical illnesses, such as heart disease predisposing to cardiotoxicity of tricyclic antidepressants. There is also an association between the occurrence of adverse reactions and the number of drugs prescribed.

Relating Effects to Drug

An effect that occurs during treatment is not necessarily due to the drug. It might be a symptom of the illness, a withdrawal effect of a recently discontinued drug or a product of suggestion due to the doctor's over-enthusiastic enquiry about unwanted effects. An effect is more likely to be due to a drug: (i) if it differs from the symptoms of the illness being treated or of any concurrent disorder; (ii) when the interval between beginning of treatment and appearance of effect makes sense in pharmacological terms; (iii) especially when the effect reappears if the drug is re-introduced.

Behavioural Effects

All psychotropic drugs influence higher cerebral function. The effects may be clinically recognisable or only discernible by refined tests of psychomotor function. Untoward effects are more likely to occur when the drug is first prescribed, when the dose is increased, when the drug is taken in large quantities, and when it is taken with other CNS depressants, including alcohol. They are particularly prone to occur in patients whose brain function is already impaired. The elderly are especially vulnerable, not only because of cerebral impairment, but also because of reduced hepatic and renal function.

The most common adverse effect is over-sedation. The patient may be drowsy with impairment of concentration, memory, intellectual functioning and performance. Such phenomena may persist for a while after treatment has been discontinued. More severe, though much less frequent, effects include confusional or delirious states.

Impairment shown on tests of complex skills suggest that psychotropic drugs may have adverse effects on driving and working with industrial machinery. Many people drive without knowing that their drugs affect their driving, and only a minority of patients are told this by their doctors. Practitioners should therefore warn patients of the dangers of driving while taking drugs.

Effects on the Fetus and Neonate

The limited research carried out in humans has not shown that the risk of dysmorphogenesis is particularly high with psychotropic drugs, but they should be avoided in pregnancy whenever possible, especially in the first trimester. The neonate may be affected by psychotropic drugs received via the placenta or breast milk. Babies are susceptible because of deficiency of drug metabolising enzymes, low protein binding and greater permeability of the blood–brain barrier.

DRUG TREATMENT OF ANXIETY

A wide variety of drugs has been used to treat anxiety. They include antidepressants such as doxepin and neuroleptics such as trifluoperazine, haloperidol, chlorpromazine and thioridazine in small doses. The use of barbiturates as anxiolytics has been abandoned. Beta-adrenoceptor blocking agents, especially propranolol, are used to treat autonomic manifestations of anxiety such as tremor or palpitations.

The most widely used drugs are the benzodiazepines. There is no convincing evidence that any one benzodiazepine is more effective than another either in relieving anxiety or inducing sleep, although there are differences in the duration of action (Table 13.2).

Diazepam is the most commonly prescribed of all antianxiety drugs. It is usually taken orally,

Table 13.2

Benzodiazepines

Duration of action	Drug	Usual daily dosage (mg)
Long – plasma half-life of drug and active metabolites over 10 hours	Chlordiazepoxide	15–30
	Clobazam	10–30
	Clorazepate	15–30
	Diazepam	4–15
	Flurazepam*	15–30†
	Ketazolam	15–60
	Medazepam	15–30
	Nitrazepam*	5–10†
Short – plasma half-life less than 10 hours	Lorazepam	2–10
	Oxazepam	30–60
	Temazepam*	10–30†
	Triazolam*	0·25†

* Marketed as a hypnotic.
† Hypnotic dose.

although it can also be given intravenously, provided resuscitative equipment is available in case of respiratory arrest. Absorption after intramuscular injection is slow and variable. Oral diazepam is rapidly absorbed and reaches a maximum blood concentration in about an hour. The plasma half-life in young adults is about 32 hours, but much longer in the elderly.

Diazepam is metabolised to N-desmethyldiazepam (nordiazepam) and then to oxazepam, both of which have therapeutic activity, before conjugation with glucuronic acid and excretion. Desmethyldiazepam has a half-life of 50–120 hours and therefore accumulates to reach concentrations greater than that of diazepam itself. There is considerable individual variation in peak steady-state plasma concentrations of diazepam, desmethyldiazepam and the ratio between the two. The metabolic pathways of diazepam and other benzodiazepines is shown in Fig. 13.2; two of diazepam's metabolites, oxazepam and clorazepate, are sold as antianxiety drugs.

Benzodiazepines bind to specific sites in the brain called benzodiazepine receptors. It is likely that the drugs are similar to an endogenous anxiolytic substance which is normally linked to these receptors.

The total clinical effect of an antianxiety drug is the sum of its pharmacological and placebo effects. The latter vary with the patient, the disorder being treated, the milieu and the drug. The placebo effect is greater in the treatment of anxiety than in the treatment of the major psychoses.

The amount of diazepam required varies widely, and in any individual one should aim at giving the lowest dose possible. Most patients require between 4 and 15 mg a day. This may be given in divided doses or as a single dose at night. Benzodiazepines should be prescribed for as short a time as possible; giving them regularly for longer than four to six weeks will probably confer little benefit. Relief from acute anxiety is usually rapid. If the patient does not respond to one

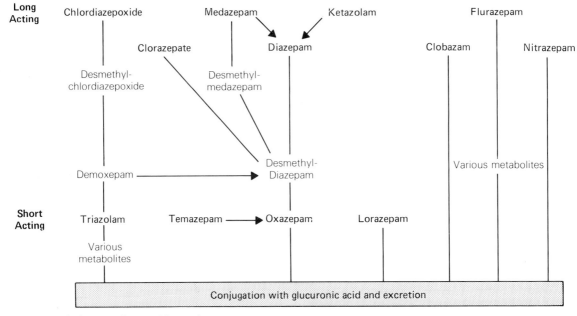

Fig. 13.2 *Metabolic interrelations of benzodiazepines.*

benzodiazepine there is no point in changing to another. The benefits of continuing treatment in chronic anxiety states are questionable. Such patients should be instructed to confine the drug to emergency use, taking it when anxiety is severe and not in regular fixed dosage.

Unwanted Effects of Benzodiazepines

Benzodiazepines seldom cause clinical problems, but dependence on them is more frequent than previously realised. Tolerance develops, although the need to increase the dose is less than with other drugs of addiction. Discontinuing treatment may cause withdrawal symptoms such as anxiety, restlessness, insomnia, tremor, and tachycardia. In rare severe cases delirium and convulsions occur. Withdrawal symptoms mostly occur within a day or two of stopping treatment, but can be delayed for several days if an active metabolite with a long duration of action is present. They last for varying periods up to ten days.

Unwanted effects during treatment are rarely severe. They include drowsiness, giddiness and, in larger doses, nystagmus, dysarthria and ataxia. Benzodiazepines cause slight respiratory depression and should be avoided if there is any danger of respiratory failure. Otherwise they are very safe even when taken in huge doses.

Diazepam taken before delivery can produce respiratory depression with bouts of apnoea, reluctance to feed and poor sucking in the neonate. Excreted in breast milk it can cause lethargy and weight loss in babies. The newborn babies of mothers taking benzodiazepines may experience withdrawal symptoms such as irritability, tremor, and tachypnoea.

The most important drug interaction is the enhancement by benzodiazepines of the depressant effects of alcohol and of the sedative effects of other psychotropic drugs.

DRUG TREATMENT OF DEPRESSION

Tricyclic and Related Drugs

The most frequently prescribed antidepressants

are the tricyclics (so-called because of their three-ring chemical structure), especially amitriptyline. Because of the tricyclics' toxicity in overdosage, some psychiatrists recommend the newer tricyclic-related antidepressants, which in general have few autonomic and cardiotoxic effects. However, less is known about the long-term effects of the newer compounds, while the main dangers of tricyclics result from faulty prescribing, especially for unhappy people liable to take overdoses (Table 13.3).

Amitriptyline is given by mouth. It is rapidly absorbed from the gut and metabolised in the liver (25–75% by first pass metabolism). Its desmethylated metabolite, nortriptyline, also has antidepressant effects. There are large genetically determined differences in metabolism of amitriptyline, leading to substantial differences in steady-state plasma concentration in different patients.

Table 13.3
Antidepressant Drugs

Type	Drug	Usual daily dosage (mg)
Tricyclics	Amitriptyline*	75–200
	Clomipramine	75–150
	Desipramine	75–200
	Dothiepin*	75–150
	Doxepin*	150–300
	Imipramine	75–200
	Nortriptyline	75–150
	Protriptyline	30–60
	Trimipramine*	75–150
Newer tricyclic-related drugs	Maprotiline*†	75–200
	Mianserin*†	60–200
	Nomifensin†	75–200
	Trazodone*†	150–300
	Zimelidine†	200–300
Monoamine oxidase inhibitors	Isocarboxazid	30–40
	Phenelzine	45–60
	Tranylcypromine	20–30
Thioxanthene	Flupenthixol	2–3

* Notable sedative properties.
† Less anticholinergic and cardiac effects.

Different investigators have found different relationships between plasma concentrations of tricyclic antidepressants and therapeutic response. There is some evidence for a poor response at low and high plasma levels and a good response in the 'therapeutic window' between – in the case of amitriptyline, at concentrations ranging from 160 to 240 ng/ml.

The plasma half-life of amitriptyline is 15 ± 5 hours. Steady-state concentrations are obtained in about a week. The active metabolite, nortriptyline, may reach higher concentrations than the parent drug itself.

Tricyclic antidepressants potentiate the action of monoamines, noradrenaline and serotonin, by inhibition of their major means of physiological inactivation – re-uptake into nerve terminals (Fig. 13.3).

Some drugs – for example, zimelidine – inhibit specifically the re-uptake of serotonin; while others – such as desipramine – block more selectively noradrenaline re-uptake. However, several newer antidepressants do not block monoamine re-uptake. Furthermore, inhibition of re-uptake is immediate, yet clinical response is delayed. The fundamental pharmacological effect, a delayed one, may be decreased sensitivity of adrenoceptors ('down-regulation').

Because of its unwanted effects, the starting dose of amitriptyline should be low, 50–75 mg a day, 25–50 mg in the elderly. This is best given in a single dose at night, when sedative and anticholinergic effects are less troublesome. The amount prescribed should be gradually increased to a maximum of 225 mg a day, 300 mg or more in exceptional cases. A dose of 150 mg daily is often effective. The rate of increase in dose should be determined by the therapeutic response and tolerance, but in most cases the dose can be doubled within a week. Elderly patients should be given lower doses. Patients should be kept on the maximum therapeutic dose tolerated for at least three or four weeks before their response can be fully assessed.

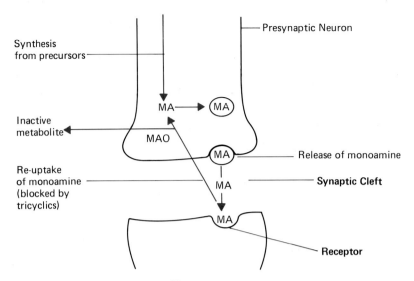

Fig. 13.3 *Diagram of a monoaminergic nerve terminal.* MA *is monoamine within a storage vesicle. MA = monoamine. MAO = monoamine oxidase.*

If the patient responds satisfactorily, there are no hard and fast rules to how long treatment should continue. Continuing maintenance treatment (about half the therapeutic dose) for six months has been shown to reduce the risk of relapse. A patient whose depression rapidly recurs when antidepressants are stopped may need continued treatment for two or more years. In general, however, those needing antidepressants for longer than six to eight months should be the exception, and there should be clear reasons for treatment to continue longer.

If the patient does not respond to treatment, one should ensure that he is taking the drug in adequate dosage. Reasons for non-compliance include unacceptable side effects and the failure by doctors to explain the aims and effects of treatment. Another reason for poor response is unusually rapid metabolism, which may be constitutionally determined or due to enzyme-inducing drugs. Accelerated metabolism may be suspected by the absence of side effects, but can only be established by estimating the plasma concentration of the drug. Once the drug has been proved ineffective, it should be discontinued.

The same principles apply to the use of all the other tricyclic and related drugs. If amitriptyline, for example, causes too much drowsiness, a less sedative drug such as despramine may be used. If a patient cannot tolerate other unwanted effects of a tricyclic, one of the newer drugs can be used.

Unwanted effects of tricyclic antidepressants

Most of these are due to the drugs' anticholinergic properties – dry mouth, sweating, tremor, blurred vision, constipation and (in patients with enlarged prostrate) urinary retention. Postural hypotension sometimes occurs.

Cardiac effects may be serious in patients with pre-existing heart disease, in whom the newer, less cardiotoxic drugs are to be preferred. Tricyclics sometimes produce ECG changes (prolonged QT interval, depressed ST segment, flattened T waves) and occasionally cause arrhythmias and even sudden death.

Central effects include the precipitation of convulsions in patients with a low seizure threshold and the stimulation of appetite, which may lead to considerable and distressing weight gain. There is evidence that tricyclics may precipitate mania in bipolar patients.

The most important drug interaction is with the antihypertensive drugs (guanethidine, bethanidine, debrisoquine) that act after uptake into the adrenergic neurone. Tricyclics decrease or abolish their uptake, thus diminishing or even reversing their hypotensive effect. Tricyclics also enhance the pressor effects of noradrenaline and adrenaline, an important consideration in local anaesthesia.

Monoamine Oxidase Inhibitors (MAOI)

The enzyme monoamine oxidase (MAO) exists in two forms, A and B. MAO-A is particularly effective in metabolising noradrenaline, dopamine and serotonin; MAO-B is more effective in the oxidation of other monoamines. Drugs that selectively inhibit either the A or the B form of the enzyme have been developed, but their usefulness in psychiatric treatment has yet to be determined. The MAOIs used in psychiatry produce maximum inhibition of both A and B forms within five to ten days. Inhibition is irreversible and normal enzyme activity can only be achieved by re-synthesis, which can take up to three weeks. Inhibition of MAO leads to the accumulation of free monoamines within neurones, thereby presumably increasing their concentration at receptor sites. Their mode of action, however, is probably much more complex.

The indications for the use of these drugs are discussed in Chapters 5 and 6. The most thoroughly investigated MAOI is phenelzine. This is given by mouth in doses of 30–60 mg daily, either in a single morning dose or in two doses after breakfast and lunch (to avoid possible initial insomnia). If there is no response and side effects are not severe, the dose may be increased up to 90 mg daily. The patient should not be regarded as unresponsive until the MAOI has been given in full dosage for four to six weeks.

In addition to the relief of depression or anxiety, some patients describe an increase in confidence, assertiveness and energy, as if the drug was exerting an amphetamine-like effect.

Because of the possible interactions (see below), patients must be instructed about dietary restrictions and other precautions. Provided the patient can be relied upon to follow the instructions, MAOIs are reasonably safe drugs. An interval of two to three weeks must be allowed after the end of treatment before the restrictions are relaxed.

Unwanted effects of MAOIs

Monoamine oxidase inhibitors have anticholinergic properties which lead to similar, but usually milder, effects to those seen with tricyclics. Postural hypotension may be a problem with large doses. Central effects include drowsiness (especially early in treatment), paradoxical difficulty in getting off to sleep, increased appetite leading to weight gain. After prolonged treatment occasional patients complain of an unpleasant 'driven' feeling – they go to bed late, feel compelled to be always active and so on.

Because of the inhibition of MAO, a large number of drug interactions may occur, of which the most important are:

(i) Indirectly acting sympathomimetic drugs (which are often a constituent of 'cold cures') have increased central and peripheral effects.

(ii) Tyramine or dopa, normally broken down by MAO in the gut mucosa and the liver, may cause hypertensive crises with, at best, a very severe pounding headache. Tyramine is present in cheese, pickled herrings, yeast extracts, any food which has undergone partial decomposition (like hung game), and certain red wines. Dopa is present in broad bean pods. The cheese reaction, as it is called, is treated with intravenous phentolamine.

(iii) Narcotics. Central effects, especially of pethidine, are prolonged. Central excitation may also occur.

(iv) Tricyclic antidepressants should not be combined with MAOIs (except in special circumstances) because their effects might be potentiated. If treatment with an MAOI is to be followed by a tricyclic, an interval of two to three weeks should be allowed.

(v) Other drugs. MAOIs potentiate antidiabetic drugs and also the depressant effects of alcohol. There may also be interactions with antihypertensive drugs.

Combined Antidepressants

Occasional patients with intractible depression seem to improve when treated with a combination of an MAOI such as phenelzine by day and a sedative tricyclic such as trimipramine at night. Such treatment should be prescribed only by experienced psychiatrists.

DRUG TREATMENT OF MANIA

Management of the Acute Episode

Mania usually calls for immediate treatment. Acute episodes can be treated with a variety of neuroleptic drugs, but haloperidol is most commonly used. Haloperidol is mostly administered orally, although it can be given intramuscularly or intravenously when a rapid effect is needed. Its mode of action is thought to be by dopamine receptor blockade and possibly adrenoceptor blockade. Haloperidol is prescribed in a starting dose of 10–30 mg a day as a single dose or in divided doses. It reduces excitement and psychomotor hyperactivity within days, although elation and grandiose ideas take longer to respond. If improvement does not occur rapidly, larger doses – up to 120 mg or more a day – may be used. When control over the symptoms is achieved, the dose should be reduced gradually to the lowest capable of maintaining improvement.

There are no hard and fast rules about the duration of treatment. As a guideline, first attacks of mania require treatment for three to six months, while second or later attacks, especially if recurring rapidly on cessation of treatment, need drugs for at least a year after hypomanic features have disappeared.

The unwanted effects of haloperidol are similar to those of other neuroleptic drugs (p.127). Mania also responds to lithium carbonate, but this takes about ten days to produce a significant effect (p. 51). Lithium and haloperidol are sometimes used together, but the combination may be dangerous, very occasionally causing brain damage with doses of haloperidol of more than 20 mg daily.

Prophylactic Treatment

Patients who have recurrent episodes of mania and/or major depression may benefit from prophylactic treatment with lithium. Lithium is rapidly and almost completely absorbed from the gastrointestinal tract. Peak plasma concentrations show a two-fold individual variation and occur 30 minutes to four hours after an oral dose. More than 95% is excreted by the kidney, while small amounts are found in saliva and in sweat. Renal clearance of lithium correlates with renal creatinine clearance. Relatively high concentrations occur in the distal and collecting tubules following peaks in serum concentration. The elimination half-life of lithium shows marked individual variation, and ranges from 7 to 20 hours. It is much more prolonged in patients with impaired renal function. Steady-state concentrations are obtained in subjects with normal renal function in two to six days.

The mode of action of lithium is not known; nor

is it known which, if any, of its many properties are relevant to its therapeutic effect.

Because lithium has a narrow therapeutic:toxic ratio, serum lithium levels should be carefully monitored. Early in treatment estimations should be carried out weekly, but when a steady-state has been achieved they need only be carried out every 2–3 months, though more often if the patient shows signs of toxicity or has a condition likely to disturb electrolyte balance. Remember that thiazide diuretics reduce renal clearance of lithium and therefore increase its plasma concentration. Estimations should also be carried out more often during pregnancy, the puerperium and breast feeding. Blood samples should be collected 12 hours after the last dose of lithium and the dose adjusted to maintain levels in the range 0·5–1·0 mmol/l.

Thyroid and renal function tests should be carried out annually. Lithium is often given as a single dose at night, but recently it has been suggested that divided doses, by reducing peak blood levels, lessen the risk of renal damage.

Lithium should be continued until the patient has been free from affective episodes for a length of time significantly exceeding the intervals between previous attacks, and very often a good deal longer. Before discontinuing treatment one should be guided by the severity of previous episodes. If, for example, the patient showed only mild flight of ideas and overactivity during previous attacks, lithium can be discontinued with more confidence than if the patient had behaved dangerously.

Unwanted effects of lithium

The unwanted effects of lithium are shown in Table 13.4. Because of the more serious of these effects, the dose of lithium should be reduced if toxic symptoms or signs appear, regardless of the serum level of lithium. Patients should be warned about the symptoms of impending toxicity.

Table 13.4
Unwanted Effects of Lithium

Effects at lower serum lithium concentration:
gastrointestinal upsets (anorexia, nausea, diarrhoea)
fine tremor (controlled by beta-blockers)
polyuria, polydipsia
oedema
weight gain

Toxic effects at higher serum lithium concentration:
restlessness
drowsiness
blurred vision
coarse tremor
ataxia, nystagmus, dysarthria

Progressing to:
delirium
convulsions
coma

Longer term effects:
non-toxic goitre
hypothyroidism
nephrogenic diabetes insipidus
focal nephron atrophy

DRUG TREATMENT OF SCHIZOPHRENIA

All acute and chronic schizophrenic patients should be given the benefit of a trial of treatment with at least one neuroleptic drug, though not all patients will need to continue with this treatment. The more commonly used drugs are shown in Table 13.5. The crucial pharmacological action of these drugs is thought to be dopamine receptor blockade.

Chlorpromazine is the most extensively investigated and most widely used of these drugs. It is mostly administered orally, but is often given intramuscularly to calm disturbed patients. Intravenous injection may cause very severe unwanted effects. It is readily absorbed from the gastrointestinal tract and reaches peak plasma levels one and a half to three hours after administration. Because of different genetically determined patterns of metabolism, there may be a fifty-fold interindividual variation in plasma levels. Even after a steady-state has been reached, individuals show a five- to ten-fold diurnal variation in concentrations. When chlorpromazine is given intramuscularly, availability increases greatly and plasma concentrations three to four

---

Table 13.5

Commonly Used Neuroleptic Drugs

Type	Drug	Usual daily dose (mg)
Phenothiazines	Chlorpromazine	150–1000
	Thioridazine	150–600
	Trifluoperazine	10–45
	Fluphenazine decanoate†	25–100*
Butyrophenones	Droperidol	20–80
	Haloperidol	10–80
Thioxanthenes	Clopenthixol decanoate†	200–400*
	Flupenthixol decanoate†	40–100*
Diphenylbutyl-piperidines	Pimozide	2–20
	Fluspirilene†	2–20**

† Depot preparation.
* Every 1–4 weeks.
** Weekly.

---

times higher than those reached by oral administration are rapidly obtained. Monitoring of plasma concentration is of little or no use in clinical practice.

Chlorpromazine is rapidly and widely distributed through the body and is highly protein-bound. It is mainly metabolised in the liver, but its metabolism is very complicated and ill understood. Some of its metabolites are therapeutically active. Its rate of elimination varies widely. Although the plasma half-life is only about six hours, chlorpromazine remains bound to tissues for long periods and metabolites are excreted for up to six months after treatment has been stopped.

Management of the Acute Episode

Treatment should begin with 200–300 mg of chlorpromazine a day or the equivalent dose of another neuroleptic. Severely disturbed patients may need considerably more than this – up to 1500 mg or more a day. In general, however, large doses should be avoided and in exceptional cases haloperidol is a safer drug to be used in large quantities. The starting dose should be increased if there is poor response, decreased when unwanted effects are troublesome. Initially the antipsychotic drug may need to be given in daily divided doses, but when the patient's condition has been stabilised it can be given as a single daily dose.

Control over psychomotor disturbance is more rapidly achieved than improvement in thought disorder, delusions and hallucinations, which may take up to six weeks to respond. A patient should not be regarded as unresponsive to a neuroleptic until it has been given in an adequate dose for this length of time. If there is no response, possible causes should be investigated. If it is thought that the patient has not been taking or absorbing the drug, an intramuscular preparation should be tried. If the patient is unresponsive to chlorpromazine, a non-phenothiazine drug, such as haloperidol, should be tried. There is no point in changing to a drug of the same category, except to reduce unwanted effects. (For example, trifluoperazine causes less drowsiness than chlorpromazine.)

Newly presenting chronic schizophrenic patients, especially those with severe negative symptoms (see p.36), respond less satisfactorily to drug treatment, but should be given the benefit of an empirical trial with one or more antipsychotic drugs. If there is then no response after three to six months treatment should be stopped.

Longer Term Management

After successful treatment of an acute episode, longer term management should be planned. If the patient can be relied on to take oral medication, chlorpromazine can be given in a single dose at night. Typical maintenance doses range from 100 to 300 mg a day. If there is doubt about the patient's compliance or if the patient accepts the advantages of long-acting injections, depot neuroleptics should be prescribed. The two most widely used preparations in Britain are fluphenazine decanoate and flupenthixol decanoate. These drugs are injected intramuscularly, are slowly absorbed and metabolised, and need only be given at one to four weekly intervals.

There are no absolute rules as to how long treatment should be continued. First attacks with good prognostic features may need only about six months' treatment, while patients with a long history of recurrent episodes of severe symptoms may need to continue treatment indefinitely. Between these extremes many patients, whose illnesses have been well controlled for about two years, should be given a trial off medication, although not at a time of stress or change.

In such cases the drug should be cautiously discontinued. The patient should be carefully supervised and, wherever possible, a relative should be advised to report any hints of deterioration. Most relapses occur within three months of stopping treatment, but can be delayed for nine months or more. The patient should therefore be seen regularly for at least nine months.

If a patient relapses when taking no medication, the neuroleptic should be reintroduced and continued for a period of time longer than that of the previous remission, before a further trial off drugs. If after two or more such trials the patient again shows signs of a relapse, medication should be continued indefinitely. When attempting to stop drug treatment one should consider the social consequences of a relapse and be more cautious when these are serious.

Many patients receiving long-term treatment with an antipsychotic drug may omit their medication two or three days a week, such as at weekends, with no untoward effect. Some psychiatrists recommend longer 'drug holidays' for carefully selected patients.

Unwanted effects of neuroleptic drugs

Neuroleptic drugs have a wide range of unwanted effects. Chlorpromazine and thioridazine have marked autonomic, and particularly anticholinergic effects, and share many of the unwanted effects of the tricyclic antidepressants. Both have marked sedative effects and chlorpromazine causes cholestatic jaundice (usually early in treatment) occasionally and photosensitivity not uncommonly. Neuroleptics may also cause weight gain, galactorrhoea and reduced libido. Otherwise, the most troublesome unwanted effects are extrapyramidal (except for thioridazine). Extrapyramidal reactions include parkinsonism, with its familiar features of rigidity, akinesia and tremor; akathisia, a subjective experience of motor restlessness leading to fidgeting and an irresistible desire to pace to and fro; and dystonic reactions, tonic spasms leading to acute attacks of abnormal movements, such as tongue protrusion, oculogyric crises and retrocollis. These reactions are often misdiagnosed: akathisia as an exacerbation of the illness, and dystonic reactions as hysteria, catatonia, epilepsy and other conditions that cause unusual movements. Diagnostic difficulties arise also when patients with insidiously developing idiopathic parkinsonism are given neuroleptics; these may be erroneously incriminated as the cause of the parkinsonism.

The above effects are reversible, whereas tardive dyskinesia, which presents as choreoathetoid movements of the mouth, lips and tongue (the 'buccolingual masticatory syndrome') and extremities, is persistent and often irreversible. It occurs more often in women, older subjects and those with prior brain damage. It is thought to be due to dopamine receptor hypersensitivity in the nigrostriatal system with a relative reduction of cholinergic function.

Neuroleptic-induced parkinsonism, akathisia

and dystonia are treated with anticholinergic drugs (Table 13.6). They should not be given routinely, but only when troublesome extrapyramidal effects occur. They should not be used to treat tardive dyskinesia as they may aggravate this condition. A wide variety of drugs have been used in an attempt to treat tardive dyskinesia, but in general results are unsatisfactory.

Table 13.6

Anticholinergic Drugs Used in the Treatment of Extrapyramidal Effects of Neuroleptics

Drug	Usual daily dosage (mg)
Benzhexol	5–15
Benztropine*	0·5–6
Orphenadrine†	100–300
Procyclidine*	5–30

* May also be given i.v. or i.m.
† May also be given i.m.

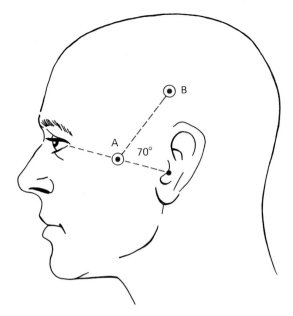

Fig. 13.4 *Electrode placement for ECT. Electrode A should be placed half-way along a line from the external angle of the eye to the external auditory meatus. Electrode B should be positioned 3 inches higher than electrode A, at an angle of 70° as indicated.*

ELECTROCONVULSIVE TREATMENT

Electroconvulsive treatment (ECT) involves the induction of a convulsion by the passage of an electric current across the brain. The current may have a sinusoidal waveform or consist of brief pulse stimuli. The electrodes are placed on the head bilaterally – anterior to the pinna of the ear – or unilaterally as shown in Fig. 13.4.

The indications for ECT in the treatment of affective disorders have been considered in Chapter 5. Electroconvulsive treatment may be helpful in severe mania that has not responded to drug treatment. Its value in schizophrenia is less certain, although it may have a part to play in the management of severe acute attacks that respond poorly to drugs. It has nothing to offer chronic schizophrenic patients. Numerous theories have been proposed to explain the mode of action of ECT, but, whatever the mechanism, the convulsion is crucial. Animal experiments suggest that this causes changes in monoamine receptor sensitivity.

Electroconvulsive treatment is given under general anaesthesia and after the administration of a muscle relaxant and atropine. Treatments are usually given either two or three times a week. The number required varies from patient to patient, most needing between two and twelve treatments, the majority four to eight. If there is no improvement at all after six to eight treatments, it is unlikely that the patient will respond to more. After optimum improvement has occurred, there is no advantage in giving one or two 'extra treatments'.

Raised intracranial pressure is the only absolute contraindication to ECT, because of the short-lived increase in cerebral blood flow that it causes. If the patient has had a recent myocardial infarct, treatment should be avoided or postponed because of the transient increase in systolic blood pressure that occurs. It should also be avoided wherever possible in patients who have cerebral or aortic aneurysms and in those who have had a cerebral haemorrhage. Treatment should be postponed if the patient has an acute respiratory infection. Electroconvulsive treatment is not contraindicated in frail elderly patients, pregnancy, or in patients with a cardiac pacemaker, spinal disease or recent fracture of long bones.

Serious complications of ECT are rare. Deaths due to ventricular arrhythmia have been reported rarely, but the risk is lower than the risk of suicide from untreated depression. Fractures and dislocations of the mid-thoracic vertebrae are hardly ever encountered since the regular use of relaxants.

Headache and post-ictal confusion are common for an hour or two after treatment. Short-term retrograde amnesia and a temporary defect in new learning also occur. These are less with unilateral ECT administered to the non-dominant hemisphere and when treatments are adequately spaced.

Some patients complain of permanent impairment of memory for past events and difficulty retaining new memories. In at least some cases, subjective complaints have not been confirmed by objective tests, and it is possible that the short-term amnesia caused by ECT draws attention to pre-existing memory impairment, including that caused by depression. The complaint is much commoner in patients who have responded poorly to ECT.

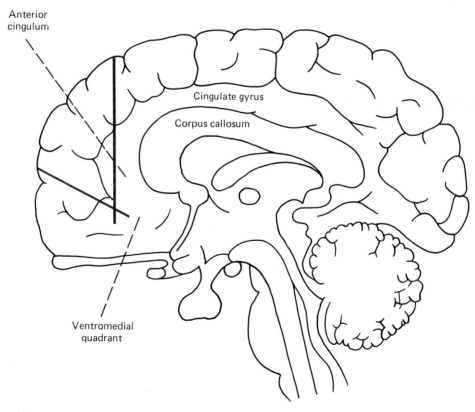

Anterior cingulum

Cingulate gyrus

Corpus callosum

Ventromedial quadrant

Fig. 13.5 *Site of lesions in psychosurgery.*

PSYCHOSURGERY

In the past, some patients with severe depressive illnesses, anxiety states, obsessional illnesses, or schizophrenia unresponsive to other treatments underwent prefrontal leucotomy. This involved freehand cutting and the surgical lesions were large. There was much post-operative morbidity due to personality deterioration and epilepsy and many patients did not improve.

As a result, prefrontal leucotomy has become obsolete and superseded by stereotactic operations. These include subcaudate tractotomy and limbic leucotomy with lesions in the cingulate area and ventromedial quadrant of the frontal lobe (Fig. 13.5). It is claimed that these techniques relieve the anguish and suffering of patients with severe affective and obsessional disorders unresponsive to all other forms of treatment. Unwanted sequelae are rare and personality deterioration is no longer encountered. There are few absolute contraindications and the operation can be carried out in old age. However, it should not be carried out in patients with marked hysterical and antisocial personality traits as they respond poorly.

Despite these encouraging claims, few patients are referred for psychosurgery, because of concern over the production of a permanent brain lesion, and the lack of controlled trials showing unequivocally that the treatment is justifiable.

14

Psychiatric Disorder and the Law

The meeting of psychiatry and the law is almost invariably over the issue of responsibility. Mental disorder may impair the sufferer's responsibility for his thinking and behaviour. Any doctor, not just a psychiatrist, can be required to make a judgement about such impairment which may have legal consequences. The law in most Western countries provides for the compulsory protection and/or treatment of the mentally disordered patient, for the protection of the general public from such patients who are judged to be dangerous, and for the mitigation of the legal penalty for those mentally disordered who commit criminal offences.

MAKING MENTAL HEALTH LAWS

In Britain the law relating to the care and control of the mentally ill has, like all British law, evolved out of the common law. During the past 200 years a series of Acts of Parliament have established the basis of modern mental health law. Concern for the mentally ill grew out of the ferment of revolutionary and humanitarian ideas that developed in the late eighteenth century. One result was the County Asylums Act of 1808, 'for the better care and maintenance of lunatics ... in England', which ultimately led to the building of our network of mental hospitals. A series of Acts dealing with the control of mental hospitals culminated in the Lunacy Act of 1890. This Act had unfortunate effects because it stipulated that admission required both a magistrate's order and clear evidence of insanity, thus preventing the in-patient treatment of early cases of good prognosis.

It was not until the Mental Treatment Act of 1930 that a patient could be admitted voluntarily. By 1952 about 70% of all admissions were voluntary. Even so, a voluntary patient could not discharge himself legally without 72 hours written notice. In 1954 a Royal Commission was set up to enquire into legal aspects of mental disorder. Most of the recommendations of their report were incorporated in the Mental Health Act (MHA) 1959 of England and Wales, which still underpins most contemporary mental health legislation. Scottish and Ulster versions of this Act were introduced in 1960 and 1961, respectively. The most important aim of this legislation was that, as far as possible, people suffering from mental disorder should be treated in the same way as those suffering from physical illnesses. In an attempt to further this aim, a series of Government White Papers was issued, each dealing with the provision of treatment facilities. In 1975 *Better Services for the Mentally Ill* urged the development of general hospital psychiatric units, with appropriate community facilities, as the eventual replacement of the large mental hospitals. In the same year the Butler Committee reported on the treatment of mentally abnormal offenders.

Since the mid-1950s the number of occupied beds in mental hospitals has fallen considerably. It has been argued that this reflects a shift of patients to reception centres and prisons rather than to the community facilities envisaged by the Department of Health. However, general psychiatric units have become increasingly important treatment centres, sometimes with good community facilities. In 1978 nearly 90% of admissions for mental disorder were informal; only 5% of in-patients at any one time were compulsorily detained. The Mental Health (Amendment) Act 1982 (MH(A)A 1982) has released informal in-patients from the few remaining legal restrictions, such as the withholding of their mail. Some are now also entitled to vote. Otherwise, it is largely concerned with the legal rights of detained patients. The changes reformed the MHA 1959 to become the MHA 1983, taking effect from September 1983.

MENTAL DISORDER DEFINED

The legal definition of mental disorder within the Mental Health Acts is vague, incorporating 'mental illness, arrested or incomplete development of mind, psychopathic disorder and any other disorder or disability of mind'. No attempt is made to define mental illness. The other three categories, severe mental impairment, mental impairment (which in the MHA 1959 were known as severe subnormality and subnormality, respectively), and psychopathic disorder are defined, with the emphasis on the social disabilities of the patient.

Many people find it illogical that mentally subnormal people, who are not actually mentally ill, should be subject to mental health legislation, while the concept of psychopathic disorder is by no means universally accepted. In the MHA 1983 it is defined as 'a persistent disorder or disability of mind (whether or not including subnormality of intelligence) which results in abnormally aggres-

sive or seriously irresponsible conduct on the part of the person concerned'.

ADMITTING PSYCHIATRIC PATIENTS TO HOSPITAL

It is worth emphasising that the overwhelming majority of those requiring treatment in Britain present as willing patients or are quite easily persuaded to accept admission to hospital. For those who are not willing, two fundamental conditions must always be met for compulsory admission. First, that mental disorder within the meaning of the Act is present and, secondly, that the person 'ought to be detained in the interests of his own health or safety or with a view to the protection of others'.

Compulsory Admissions in an Emergency

When a patient is acutely disturbed and refuses hospital admission, it ought not to be difficult to find people who may legally sanction a short hospital admission to allow more detailed planning of care to take place in safety. For the emergency provisions (summarised in Table 14.1), therefore, very few restrictions are placed on the class of person who may authorise detention. The variations chiefly arise because patients may be involved in crisis in a variety of places. The emergency system has been criticised on two counts: it may lead to the unnecessary detention of patients who have no rights of appeal against these orders, yet at the same time it does not always allow sufficiently rapid action. A new provision (section 5, MHA 1983) attempts to deal in part with the latter problem by allowing 'prescribed' nursing staff to detain informal in-patients for up to six hours.

Table 14.1

Compulsory Emergency Admissions

Section of MHA	Signatures required	Place of patient at presentation	Place receiving patient	Maximum detention time allowed
4	Nearest relative or social worker + Any doctor	Not specified	Hospital	72 hours
135	Magistrate	Home (allows powers of entry)	'Place of safety' (usually hospital)	72 hours
136	Police officer	Public place	'Place of safety'	72 hours
5	Doctor in charge of patient's care	Hospital	Hospital	72 hours
	Nurse of prescribed class	Hospital	Hospital	6 hours

Planned Compulsory Admissions

Greater safeguards exist for patients compulsorily admitted for longer periods. The important conditions for imposing these orders are summarised in Table 14.2. In the case of sections 2 and 3 the nearest available relative should be involved in the application even if this is finally made by the social worker. One of the doctors must be recognised by the local Health Authority as having special experience in the management of mental disorder. Although most patients are subsequently discharged from compulsory treatment when their doctors consider them to be improved or recovered, some patients wish to challenge their detention sooner. Patients in both categories may apply to the managers of the hospital where they are detained or to an independent Mental Health Review Tribunal (MHRT) for a formal examination of their case with a view to discharge from the order. The tribunal consists of lawyers, doctors and lay people, the latter usually with special knowledge or experience of social services. It hears evidence from the patient or his representative as well as from the doctor who wishes the patient to continue to be detained. It may order the patient's discharge.

Other Aspects of Civil Law in Relation to the Psychiatric Patient

The MHA provides for the protection and management of the property as well as the person of the mentally disordered. Under section 94 of the MHA, medical evidence may be offered that any form of mental disorder renders a person incapable of managing his property and affairs. This is put to a judge in a special court – The Court of Protection – who, if satisfied, may then appoint a Receiver to act on behalf of the patient and keep his accounts. The Receiver may be a relative or friend, although in many cases a solicitor, bank trustee or Official Solicitor of the Supreme Court takes this role. The patient and his affairs may be checked from time to time by medical and legal 'Visitors' appointed by the Lord Chancellor. Medical Visitors must have special knowledge and experience of mental disorder.

Another problem may be the validity of a

Table 14.2

Compulsory Admissions: Intermediate and Long Term

	Section of MHA	Exclusion criteria by diagnosis	Signatures required	Maximum detention time allowed
	2	None	Nearest relative or social worker + Two doctors	28 days
	3	Mental impairment or psychopathic disorder if treatment unlikely to be effective	Nearest relative or social worker + Two doctors	6 months
From the Criminal Courts	37	None	Any court (conviction not invariable) + Two doctors	6 months
	41	None	Higher court only (conviction essential) + Two doctors; at least one must give oral evidence	Any length of time greater than one year; may be indefinite
From Prison	47/48	None	Secretary of State + Two doctors	Length of prison term (earliest release date)
	49	None	Secretary of State	As section 41

person's will. A doctor may be asked, sometimes after the death of the person, whether that person possessed 'Testamentary Capacity'. In order to make a valid will a person must have been able to understand the nature of a will, to know the extent of his property and the likely extent of the claims on it *at the time of making the will.*

The other main area of civil law on which mental disorder impinges is divorce. Under the Matrimonial Causes Act 1937 insanity may be given as a reason for divorce and nullification of a marriage although the criteria are strict: the respondent must be 'incurably of unsound mind' and have been 'continuously under care and treatment for a period of at least five years immediately preceding the presentation of the petition'. At least the early part of that treatment should have been under compulsory detention.

The Mental Health Act Commission

The MHA 1983 has two completely new, important and controversial provisions. A special health authority, known as the Mental Health Act Commission, is to be set up, while consent to treatment is removed in law from the setting of the traditional doctor–patient relationship in a variety of situations. The MHA Commission will be a multidisciplinary body, which will have a general overseeing role for any aspect of psychiatric care; for example, inspecting hospital and mental nursing homes. On issues of consent to treatment, members of the Commission will advise on the Secretary of State's regulations, to be appended to the Act, and will have special roles for individual patients. If psychosurgery or 'such other treatments as may be specified . . . by the Secretary of

State' (listed in regulations issued from time to time) are proposed, one medical and two lay members of the Commission must provide a certificate sanctioning the treatment before it can proceed. The certificate is necessary even though the patient is informal, judged competent to consent and giving consent. Controls on other treatments apply only to compulsorily detained patients, and only then if the patient is withholding his consent, or judged by his own psychiatrist to be incompetent to consent. The regulations affect any courses of 'medicine' which last longer than three months but also some treatments 'specified by the Secretary of State' (at present only electro-convulsive treatment). In these cases one medical practitioner alone from the MHA Commission is required to sanction treatment.

Planned Compulsory Admission of Offender Patients

If a person has committed an offence which is punishable with imprisonment, and two doctors, one at least with special experience, are agreed that he or she is suffering from mental disorder, then either a magistrates court or a higher court may order that the person is detained in a hospital under section 37 of the MHA (see Table 14.2). In common with most orders for compulsory detention, the patient on a section 37 order has to be admitted within a fixed time of the order being made (in this case 28 days) or the order expires. The court has no powers to compel a hospital authority to receive a patient, so usually also insists on hearing that a bed is available for the person.

In most respects, such as length, powers of discharge and appeal, the section 37 order is very similar to section 3. Occasionally, when the case is dealt with entirely in a magistrates court, the magistrates may make an order under section 37 without convicting the patient, providing they are satisfied that the person did commit the offence

and could have been imprisoned if convicted. In this case, however, only mental illness or severe mental impairment are allowed as reasons for detention.

The higher courts may impose a 'restriction order', section 41, when it is thought that the patient may pose a special risk to the public. This may be imposed to restrict discharge for a fixed period, but much more commonly to restrict it indefinitely. Until the MHA 1983 discharge from a restriction order could only be ordered by the Home Secretary. Now it may also be ordered by a special MHRT, chaired by a judge, providing the tribunal is satisfied that further detention 'is not in the interest of the patient's health or safety or for the protection of other persons'. The responsible doctor has only an advisory role in discharge.

Under sections 47 and 48 the Secretary of State may order the transfer of a person from prison to hospital providing that two doctors are agreed that he suffers from any kind of mental disorder which warrants detention in hospital for treatment. An additional direction (section 49) restricting discharge may also be imposed.

THE MENTALLY ABNORMAL OFFENDER IN COURT

When a person is held on suspicion of having committed a criminal offence, he is often at the beginning of a very long ordeal. He must be charged quickly – within three days – but his trial is likely to be months in the future for all but the most trivial offences and, following that, he may have the prospect of a custodial or a socially supervised sentence stretching ahead. The offender may already have established mental disorder but each stage of the process is very stressful, be it the committing of the offence, being questioned, being held on remand, or appearing in court, and the offender may develop a psychiatric disorder at any stage. The law takes account of this. It is legally possible not only for an offender to receive treatment within the penal system but also, if necessary, for him to be transferred to an outside hospital for treatment at any stage of his remand or detention if his disorder requires this (see Table 14.3).

For most doctors working outside the prison service the critical issues arise around the offender's court appearances and requests by the court or by the offender's defence counsel to provide relevant reports about his mental state.

The court requires answers to three main questions which relate to each of the three main phases of the hearing (see Table 14.3):

1. Is the alleged offender mentally fit enough to be tried?
2. Can the alleged offender be found guilty of the offence with which he is charged in the light of his mental state at the time of the offence?
3. Should the mental state of the offender be taken into account in passing sentence?

Table 14.3

The Mentally Abnormal Offender

Stage of legal process	Time when mental disorder must have been present	Nature of plea	Medical consequences
Pre-trial	Following the offence	—	a) Informal/formal treatment on bail b) Bail conditional on treatment c) Transfer from prison to hospital (section 48) d) Remand to hospital for report or treatment (Crown Court)
Pre-trial	The time of the trial	Unfit to plead	Compulsory in-patient treatment without trial on original charge
Trial: Conviction stage	The time of the offence	a) Non-insane automatism (any charge) b) Insane (murder) c) Diminished responsibility (murder)	a) Aquittal but compulsory admission to hospital if charge serious b) Aquittal but compulsory admission to hospital c) Guilty of manslaughter. Any sentence possible
Trial: Sentencing stage	The time of the offence and/or the trial	Guilt established; mitigation on medical grounds	a) Remand to hospital for report (Magistrates Court) b) Interim hospital order (Crown Court) c) Section 37 ± section 41. Compulsory admission to hospital d) Probation order with condition of in- or out-patient treatment e) Custodial sentence with expectation of treatment in prison f) Non-custodial sentence with voluntary or compulsory (section 3) treatment
—	After sentencing	—	Treatment in prison Transfer to Special/NHS Hospital S47/49

* Under section 3, Criminal Courts Act 1973, not MHA.

Fitness to Plead

The question of fitness to plead is rarely raised. It has to be argued before a jury in a higher court and the consequences of being found unfit to plead are very serious. In general, no further examination takes place under English law, not even a trial of the facts. At worst an innocent man may find himself under lengthy detention in a mental hospital without right of appeal. Inevitably the ruling tends to be reserved for those who are very severely mentally disordered and on very serious charges. There are traditional tests of fitness to plead; the defendant should be capable of instructing counsel, appreciating the significance of pleading 'guilty' or 'not guilty', challenging a juror, examining the witnesses, understanding and following the evidence and the court procedure, but strictly the definition of someone who is unfit to plead is very simple ' . . . he is under a disability which would constitute a bar to his being tried' (Criminal Procedure Insanity Act 1964).

Establishing Guilt

The next phase of the hearing is concerned with the offence and the two issues fundamental to establishing guilt or otherwise. The first is non-medical and rests on whether it can be shown that the accused carried out the illegal act (*actus reus*), but the second requires psychiatric evidence to aid the court in deciding whether the accused intended to commit the offence (*mens rea*).

The insanity defence

In 1843, Daniel McNaughton, under the influence of paranoid delusions and in the belief that he was attacking the Prime Minister, killed his secretary. Following his trial the House of Lords established the legal criteria for a finding of 'not guilty by reason of insanity'. They ruled that it must be established that *at the time of the act* the accused's mind was so disordered or defective that he did not know the nature and quality of the act he was doing or, that if he did know this, he did not know that the act was wrong. If the defence successfully establishes insanity by these rules, no conviction is recorded against the accused, but he is invariably detained in a mental hospital under the Criminal Procedure Insanity Act 1964.

Diminished responsibility

In relation to a person charged with murder it is now far more likely that the psychiatrist will be asked a slightly different question about the accused's mental state: 'Was he suffering from such abnormality of mind as substantially impaired his mental responsibility for his acts in doing or being a party to the killing?' (Homicide Act 1957). In the Court of Appeal an 'abnormality of mind' in this Act has been established as 'a state of mind so different from that of ordinary human being's that the reasonable man would term it abnormal'. If the defence is successful in establishing diminished responsibility the conviction recorded is reduced from murder to manslaughter. Thus, the judge is released from passing the mandatory life sentence. He may still impose life imprisonment but is free to choose, for example, to order psychiatric treatment in hospital or even in the community.

An infanticide plea is, in practice, a variant of the diminished responsibility plea. (In Law, infanticide is the murder by a woman of her own child within a year of its birth.)

Automatism

Rarely various transient states may render persons unconscious of their behaviour while leaving them physically free to act, so that they cannot form the necessary intent to perform a criminal act. These include epileptic automatism, hypoglycaemia and somnambulism. The Court of Appeal has ruled that when these disturbances are secondary to long-standing disorder, such as brain damage, the patient must be regarded as insane, so that even though the individual must be found not guilty, indeterminate hospital detention under the Criminal Procedure Insanity Act 1964 should follow. Non-insane automatism is a term retained only for those states when an external agent (for example, insulin administered to a diabetic) has triggered the attack.

Sentencing

Most psychiatric evidence presented in court is for this phase of the trial. The courts vary conviction on the grounds of absent or reduced responsibility only in the circumstances described above, but they do allow impaired responsibility in other cases to be considered as an excuse when the sentencing phase is reached. They may simply reduce the penalty imposed for the offence. If psychiatric disorder remains a problem they usually accept guidance from the reporting doctor about the necessity for treatment. They may allow the offender to remain free to pursue voluntary treatment; if the offender expresses a wish for treatment but there is some doubt about his capacity for keeping up his commitment, a Probation Order with a Condition of Treatment may be imposed; compulsory detention in a mental hospital under the MHA is another possibility. If the offender is sentenced to imprisonment there is a possibility of psychiatric treatment within prison but neither judge nor magistrate may order this. There is an important special facility within the prison service; Grendon Prison is a psychiatric prison which is run, as far as Home Office rules allow, along therapeutic community lines for non-psychotic offenders.

The right to receive treatment

In recent years it has often been difficult or impossible to find a hospital bed for a mentally abnormal offender whose need for psychiatric treatment has been recognised by the court. Paradoxically the least dangerous seem most likely to be denied treatment. For those who are ill and dangerous there is another layer of health care available within the Special Hospital system. There are four such hospitals in England (e.g. Broadmoor) and one in Scotland; their administration is outside both the general NHS and the prison systems. They offer maximum security but also a predominantly medical approach to treatment. Recently a small number of Regional Secure Units have been established, usually in the grounds of a psychiatric hospital. They offer less security but a range of treatment and rehabilitation which more closely resembles that ideally available in ordinary psychiatric units.

MENTAL HEALTH LAW IN SCOTLAND

This chapter has discussed the law obtaining in England and Wales. The law in Scotland is broadly similar, but differs in at least three important details. First, the Mental Health (Scotland) Act 1960 recognises only two forms of mental disorder: mental illness and mental deficiency. Second, it requires the approval of a legal officer for planned compulsory admission. Third, it established a Mental Health Commission 'generally to exercise protective functions' in respect of mentally ill patients. The Commission can discharge patients from compulsory detention. It must also regularly visit hospitals in which patients are detained, and look into allegations of mistreatment, wrongful detention and the like.

Emergency admission, and also the detention in hospital of an informal in-patient, is permissible under section 31 (cf. sections 4 and 5 in England and Wales). There is no mechanism for admission for observation, comparable to the English section 2. However, admission for treatment, under section 24, requires a review within 28 days. This type of admission needs the approval of the nearest relative (or a Mental Health Officer) and two doctors, but also of the Sheriff. This officer also carries out the main function of the English Mental Health Review Tribunal, in that he hears appeals against detention.

The principal means of compulsory admission in Scotland are set out in Table 14.4.

At the time of writing major amendments to the Scottish Health Act were being considered.

Table 14.4

Compulsory Admission in Scotland

Section of MHA	Signatures required	Place of patient at presentation	Place receiving patient	Maximum detention allowed
31	Nearest relative or Mental Health Officer + Any doctor	In community or in hospital	Hospital	7 days
24	Nearest relative or Mental Health Officer + Two doctors + Sheriff	Not specified	Hospital	1 year (review within 28 days)
104	Police Officer	Public place	Place of safety	72 hours

15

Psychiatric Disorder and Crime

Is There a Relationship?

As crime and psychiatric disorder are both common, the two might be expected to occur together quite often by chance. It has never been established that there is a greater than chance association; it would be necessary to correlate data about psychiatric symptoms and offending behaviour in individuals from a substantial representative sample of the general population. A survey concerned with such a broad question, however, would be of little practical value.

Crime is a social concept which varies over time and between societies. Until quite recently suicide and all male homosexual behaviour were criminal offences in this country. Abuse, mutilation and even killing of children by their families was, however, largely ignored until well into this century, despite preliminary legislation on their behalf in 1889. In some States of America cohabitation is technically an offence, whereas in some tribes in India paedophilia is not only allowed in law but encouraged. Crime includes murder and robbery, but over 60% of all crimes dealt with by British courts concern motoring. Similarly, psychiatric disorder as a global concept has almost as little value as the term crime.

Given these problems of definition, a better approach to the issue is to examine whether there are special relationships between subgroups of criminals and certain kinds of mental illness. Two recent American studies suggested that

there may not be. The source of the samples seemed to have the biggest effect on the nature of the subgroups. One study examined prisoners serving sentences for a range of serious offences. Nine-tenths had a psychiatric disorder – in most cases personality disorder and/or alcohol or drug abuse; less than 1% were schizophrenic. The other study, of ex-mental hospital patients, showed a substantial arrest rate (47% over eight years) and a high association between schizophrenia and both violent and non-violent crime. Since the majority of the patients were schizophrenic this was inevitable! A third study from Germany showed that, over ten years, among those charged with serious personal violence 3% showed schizophrenia, major affective disorder or mental retardation – the same proportion as would be expected in the general population.

Another problem that prevents a reliable estimate of the relationship is that most crime is undetected and the factors that influence detection are unknown. Are the mentally ill more likely to be caught offending and so over-represented in the criminal population? Are they more likely to be excused for their behaviour at the time of detection and so under-represented? Whichever is a more potent factor, another American study confirmed that 'official crime', the key criterion in many studies, is a poor reflection of reality. Of 321 hospital admissions for mental illness 36% had been preceded by actual or threatened violence.

Only three patients in the sample had been arrested.

A substantial proportion of prisoners probably do need some psychiatric assistance and many psychiatric patients may offend. How does this arise? It is usual to look to the mental disorder to explain the crime, but the reverse possibility must not be forgotten. In a series of mentally abnormal homicides 27% had become psychotic after the killing. Crime and its consequences are stressful life events. It is also possible that some common factor may predispose both to mental disorder and criminal behaviour.

Official criminal statistics suggest that the courts are more likely to send to hospital those convicted of personal violence, sex offences, arson and other damage to property than other types of offenders. Routine psychiatric admissions, too, often follow violent behaviour. Several American studies suggest that about 10% of admissions follow attacks on other people, a similar rate to admissions after deliberate self harm. Clearly, a strategy for assessing violent and dangerous behaviour is important, whether strictly criminal or not.

ASSESSMENT OF VIOLENT BEHAVIOUR

A good approach is to regard the violent patient as rather similar to the suicidal patient. An essential question is whether, since the violent threat or act, the person's attitudes or situation have changed. If not, then the risk of further violent behaviour is high. One must also decide how damaging that behaviour is likely to be, and to whom, not forgetting that strong suicidal ideas often co-exist with externally directed aggression. A useful answer to any of these questions depends on a systematic appraisal of each major contributor to the violence: the violent person, the victim and the surroundings. A possible scheme for this is outlined in Fig. 15.1.

The Illness Related Variables

If there is no medical diagnosis, then there is no case for medical intervention, although medical limits are often harder to define than this statement suggests. Does the person who is violent in the context of occasional excessive drinking present a medical problem? Many habitually violent people acquire a label of personality disorder, which has medical respectability, but there is little evidence that medical treatment is more than occasionally helpful. Within the mentally ill group schizophrenics seem the most likely to be violent. Deluded depressed patients may kill, but violence is very rare among depressives, as it is among manics despite their often threatening stance. The role of brain damage in precipitating violence is unclear. Certainly a direct relationship remains unproven in more than a minority of cases. In America the concept of 'episodic dyscontrol' has become very popular. This explains motiveless violent outbursts by attributing them to sudden discharges, akin to epilepsy, within the limbic system of the brain. Abuse of drugs or alcohol, however, is another feature of the syndrome and might be a better explanation of the loss of control in most subjects.

Sometimes a particular symptom is important in precipitating aggressive behaviour. Paranoid delusions, particularly if the patient has already been acting on them without relief, not uncommonly culminate in violence. It seems likely that the most dangerous situation is when the delusions develop in isolation and not as part of a major psychosis. There are two reasons for this: the delusions are more likely to go unrecognised when the person is otherwise relatively normal and, because of the person's relatively intact personality and freedom from other symptoms, the violence is more likely to be effectively executed. However, much of the violent behaviour of psychotics results from the same motives that breed violence in psychiatrically normal people, e.g. a reaction to rejection.

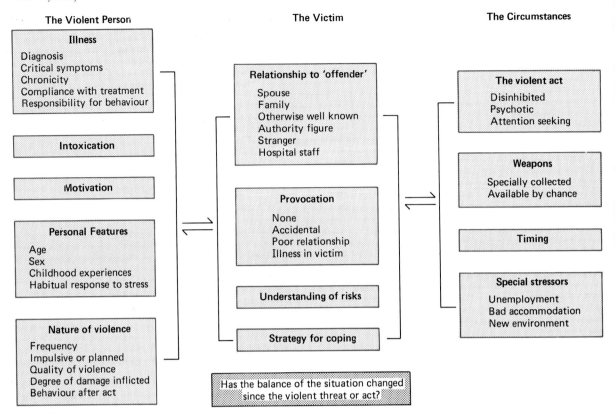

The Violent Person

Illness
Diagnosis
Critical symptoms
Chronicity
Compliance with treatment
Responsibility for behaviour

Intoxication

Motivation

Personal Features
Age
Sex
Childhood experiences
Habitual response to stress

Nature of violence
Frequency
Impulsive or planned
Quality of violence
Degree of damage inflicted
Behaviour after act

The Victim

Relationship to 'offender'
Spouse
Family
Otherwise well known
Authority figure
Stranger
Hospital staff

Provocation
None
Accidental
Poor relationship
Illness in victim

Understanding of risks

Strategy for coping

Has the balance of the situation changed since the violent threat or act?

The Circumstances

The violent act
Disinhibited
Psychotic
Attention seeking

Weapons
Specially collected
Available by chance

Timing

Special stressors
Unemployment
Bad accommodation
New environment

Fig. 15.1 *Assessment of violence.*

Although the acutely psychotic patient may be violent, there is evidence that the chronically ill patient presents a greater threat. Within the schizophrenic subsample of a substantial series of homicidal offenders 84% had been ill for over a year at the time of their offence and 55% for more than five years. Less than 3% were violent within four weeks of the onset of their psychosis. The label of 'personality disorder' by definition implies disturbance of long duration. Part of the problem may be in treatment compliance. This is probably at its poorest among the groups for whom treatment is of most doubtful value, the personality disordered. In the schizophrenic group referred to above, in the six months before the violent crime nearly 70% of the patients had received no treatment.

Perhaps the most important issue raised by mental disturbance is whether the patient is able to take responsibility for his behaviour. In the courts this is always debated after a violent act has taken place, but the same questions apply. Is the patient's perception of his actions or his surroundings impaired? Can he control his behaviour whether or not his judgement is sound?

Some Personal Features

Except among depressives, in both sick and healthy populations youth and male gender are most likely to be associated with physical violence. A history of major losses and deprivation in childhood is common, as is one of parental violence and alcohol abuse. It is generally claimed, however, that the best predictor of future violence is the nature of previous violence. Nevertheless, homicide is rarely a recidivist crime and for all forms of violence the ideal is to prevent 'the first time'. A detailed account of all threatened or actual violence, including self harm, must be collected, preferably from independent informants as well as the individual concerned. Occasionally some specific details are helpful. For example, an attack directed to a particular part of the body, such as a nose or an eye rather than the whole person, is more likely to be psychotic. After homicide suicide is very common (about a third of cases in this country), so special observations will be necessary.

The Victim

In many violent episodes the victim's role is as critical as the aggressor's. At least 25% of victims of violent or sexual crimes have been victims before. The nature of the relationships in which violence has been a factor, and their importance to the patient, must be fully assessed. Relations or close acquaintances are generally more vulnerable, but one must remember that class of relationship may be as important as actual relationship. Anyone who has, for example, taken on the wife role, or is seen by the patient to have done so, may become as vulnerable to violence as the real wife. This is as important in hospital as in the community.

Provocation by the victim may sometimes be quite deliberate, particularly in the context of a deteriorating relationship. Even among the most obviously mentally ill this problem cannot be ignored. Sometimes, however, the provocation may be accidental. For example, a gesture may be given a psychotic interpretation. Illness in the victim – mental or physical – is another factor. Many child victims of parental violence are underweight at birth, going through a developmental crisis or a minor illness at the time of abuse.

The fact that many actual and potential victims are emotionally close to the aggressor sets another problem. They often have great difficulty in understanding or acknowledging the risk to themselves, particularly if their relationship with the patient was good up to the time of onset of an illness. Pathological jealousy is a notoriously dangerous state, but although the victim is warned he, or more usually she, is generally very reluctant to separate.

The Circumstances

A psychiatric unit is inevitably a place where violence is likely to occur. Violence is often simply the expression of fear or despair in the context of illness or deteriorating personal relationships. Many patients recognise this and seek medical help for their behaviour. Many are brought by others for the same reasons. Otherwise the place where the violence occurs is often a matter of chance or of largely unrelated factors. The chronic schizophrenic, for example, may be more likely to damage public property than domestic premises, but if he is of 'no fixed abode' he has no personal property to attack. His destructiveness may be largely help-seeking behaviour. Weapons too are often available by chance rather than design. It is undoubtedly important to separate the patient and his known weapons, but this alone will not necessarily ensure safety as commitment to an idea is usually accompanied by inventiveness.

Self harm staged for early discovery is often fairly trivial and the same is true of other violent behaviour. On the whole the smashing of windows is done as the police turn the corner to watch. Occasionally, however, illnesses show predictable fluctuations in their course or a violent outburst may follow closely on an additional problem thrust on to the already overwrought patient. Awareness of recent or imminent additional stresses in the patient's life and provision of appropriate support may be critical in preventing disaster.

THE MANAGEMENT OF THE POTENTIALLY VIOLENT PATIENT

The management is already well started by an efficient and sympathetic assessment. The patient's relief at having his fears heard is not to be underestimated, even for the psychotic. Decisions follow about whether the patient needs to remain in hospital and whether his voluntary commitment to this is adequate, about instituting appropriate treatment and about organising other forms of supervision and assistance. Staff from other disciplines are ideally involved in this kind of planning.

Occasionally direct intervention during violence will be required. In the interests of safety for everyone, clear policies for this kind of management should be well known to all hospital staff. Potentially violent patients should only be seen or nursed in areas where clear observation is possible, to which other staff have rapid and easy access and where an alarm system is readily available. Obvious makeshift weapons such as heavy ashtrays must not be lying around. This approach should apply for all new and unknown patients seen in an emergency room, as well as for those with a formidable reputation. If reassurance is failing, withdrawal is better than confrontation. It is vital, for example, not to get into a conflict over trying to remove a weapon. Physical restraint may become necessary but should only be initiated when several members of staff are available. If this has happened in hospital, sedative intramuscular medication is necessary too, and this should have been prepared. Careful observations of the patient must follow and, as soon as the crisis is passed, those involved with the incident and the patient's future care must meet to discuss the incident and plan future management to prevent further incidents.

SOME SPECIAL CATEGORIES OF OFFENDER PATIENTS

Psychiatrists frequently become involved in the assessment and even management of people who have no formal mental illness and this is particularly true of offenders. We are frequently, and rightly, reminded that to confine or treat people solely because of dangerous or socially unacceptable behaviour, however good our intentions, is akin to the political abuse of psychiatry by totalitarian regimes. Delinquents, female offenders and sex offenders most often fall into this category, although a fourth group – the elderly offenders – may become more important as it grows in size.

Juvenile Delinquency

Law breaking between the ages of 10 (the age of criminal responsibility) and 21 is generally referred to as delinquency. About half of juvenile offenders commit only one offence, while in the remainder criminal behaviour usually ceases in the early 20s. Nevertheless, half of all serious crime is committed by people under the age of 21, so that delinquency is a major problem. Delinquents who continue in their criminal careers appear to be socially and emotionally deprived. That may be why psychiatric assistance is so much sought. Some factors, such as low social class, poverty and overcrowding, are not now thought to be very important. However, large families, parental discord and poor parenting behaviour (including over-indulgent, inconsistent and harsh discipline), are still thought to be important precipitants. There is often a family history of criminality, but evidence from twin studies does not support a genetic basis. Evaluation of treatment programmes has shown few positive results. 'Unsuitable candidates' for counselling seem likely to do worse than their untreated peers, but those who are bright, verbal, anxious and motivated to change may do well.

Psychopathy

The Butler Committee, commissioned by the Government to report on mentally abnormal offenders, is just one among the many groups and individuals who have recommended abandoning the term psychopath. The main arguments against the concept are: first, that its definition is circular – mental abnormality is inferred from antisocial conduct and then used to explain it; second, that it has become a pejorative term, dependent on subjective judgements, which may interfere with the individual's requests or rights to treatment; third, that there is little agreement between psychiatrists on its meaning or application; fourth, that it is of little value in predicting response to treatment.

In one study a series of men in Grendon Psychiatric Prison, diagnosed by various psychiatrists as 'psychopathic', underwent extensive research assessments. No single factor, other than their presence in this prison, identified them as psychopaths. All the men were highly motivated towards their treatment, including group psychotherapy. Their level of neurotic symptoms was high on arrival at the prison and declined during therapy. Their subsequent reconviction rate was, however, no different from that of inmates of other prisons who had had no treatment. Perhaps, in this type of prisoner, offending and symptomatology are not directly related.

Female Offenders

Although the rate of identified female crime, and particularly violent crime, seems to be rising, male offenders still outnumber female offenders by about 8:1. Female offenders arouse interest because a few offences are committed almost exclusively by women. In the case of infanticide special provision is made in law (see p.137). Offences relating to prostitution, which itself is not illegal, and child stealing are other such offences, but shoplifting is probably the most important numerically. Although this offence occurs among all ages, sexes and social classes, it is committed with unusual frequency by women over the age of 40 who, if they re-offend, tend to continue in the same pattern. Twenty per cent of female first offenders and 30% of recidivists have a psychiatric disorder, particularly depression, and 10% have a major physical illness. In most instances, however, there is little value in treating female offenders differently from their male counterparts. The one exception is concerned with the exclusively female function of menstruation. There is evidence that women are at their most vulnerable in the few days immediately around the onset of menstruation. Self harm, other forms of aggression and criminal offences all seem to be more common at this time. In two recent criminal trials a history of premenstrual tension has successfully been used as an absolute excuse for a woman's behaviour.

Sex Offenders

'Sex offender' is a collective term of little value. It encompasses everyone from the indecent exposer to the sadistic murderer. Psychiatrists have become very involved in assessment and treatment, partly because people with sexual problems tend to regard their problems as 'medical', partly because of psychoanalytic theory and partly because of the availability of libido-suppressing drugs which are only available on medical prescription (see p.107). There is, however, little evidence that any treatment, whether penal or medical, can be relied upon to modify persistently deviant sexual behaviour.

Constant and careful review of medical and psychiatric intervention in each of these categories is very important. It may be that some very useful medical contributions derive from preventive rather than clinical medicine. Doctors should pay more attention to the importance of alcohol abuse as a cause of crime, and to the importance of alcoholism prevention programmes in the prevention of crime. After all, 6% of all convictions in British courts are for drunkenness and many more offences are committed under the influence of alcohol (see Chapter 9). Medical pressure groups, along the lines of antismoking groups might, if they succeed in modifying public attitudes to alcohol, have more effect on the rates of some crimes than any other medical intervention.

Further Reading

Chapter 1

Clare A. (1976). *Psychiatry in Dissent*. London: Tavistock.

Kendell R.E. (1975). *The Role of Diagnosis in Psychiatry*. Oxford: Blackwell.

Lewis A. (1967). Health as a social concept. In: *The State of Psychiatry*. London: Routledge and Kegan Paul, pp. 179–94.

Wing J.K. (1978). *Reasoning about Madness*. Oxford: Oxford University Press.

Chapter 2

The Department of Psychiatry Teaching Committee of the Institute of Psychiatry. (1978). *Notes on Eliciting and Recording Clinical Information*. Oxford: Oxford Medical Publications.

Kahn R.L., Goldfarb A.J., Pollack M., Peck A. (1960). Brief objectives measures for the determination of mental status in the aged. *American Journal of Psychiatry*, **117**: 326–8.

Leff J.P., Isaacs A.D. (1978). *Psychiatric Examination in Clinical Practice*. Oxford: Blackwell.

Chapter 3

Lishman W.A. (1978). *Organic Psychiatry*. Oxford: Blackwell.

Lloyd G.G. (1977). Psychological reactions to physical illness. *British Journal of Hospital Medicine*, **18**: 352–68.

Chapter 4

Hamilton M. (1976). *Fish's Schizophrenia*. Bristol: John Wright and Sons.

Wing J.K., Wing L., eds (1982). *Handbook of Psychiatry 3: Psychoses of Uncertain Aetiology*. Cambridge: Cambridge University Press, Chapters 1–14.

Chapter 5

Brown G.W., Harris T.O., Copeland J.R. (1977). Depression and loss. *British Journal of Psychiatry*, **130**: 1–18.

Kendell R.E. (1976). The classification of depression: a review of contemporary confusion. *British Journal of Psychiatry*, **129**: 15–28.

Paykel E.S., Rowan P.R. (1979). Affective disorders. In: Granville-Grossman K., ed, *Recent Advances in Clinical Psychiatry, 3*. Edinburgh: Churchill Livingstone, pp. 37–90.

Roth M., Gurney C., Garside R.F., Kerr T.A. (1972). Studies in the classification of affective disorders. The relationship between anxiety states and depressive illnesses. *British Journal of Psychiatry*, **121**: 147–61.

Chapter 6

Chodoff P. (1974). The diagnosis of hysteria. *American Journal of Psychiatry*, **131**: 1073–8.

Lader M. (1972). The nature of anxiety. *British Journal of Psychiatry*, **121**: 481–91.

Marks I.M. (1973). Research in neurosis: a selective review. 1. Causes and courses. *Psychological Medicine*, **3**: 436–54.

Merskey H. (1978). Hysterical phenomena. *British Journal of Hospital Medicine*, **19**: 305–9.

Snaith P. (1981). *Clinical Neurosis*. Oxford: Oxford University Press.

Chapter 7

Jacoby R.J. (1981). Depression in the elderly. *British Journal of Hospital Medicine*, **25**: 40–7.

Jeffery P.M., Jacoby R., Murray R. (1979). The psychiatry of old age: 1 General principles and functional disorders. In: Hill P., Murray R., Thorley A., eds, *Essentials of Postgraduate Psychiatry*. London: Academic Press, pp. 473–89.

Lishman W.A. (1978). Senile dementia, presenile dementia and pseudomentia. In: *Organic Psychiatry*. Oxford: Blackwell, pp. 527–94.

Pitt B. (1982). *Psychogeriatrics: An Introduction to the Psychiatry of Old Age*, 2nd ed. Edinburgh: Churchill Livingstone.

Chapter 8

Farmer R.D.T., Hirsch S.R., eds (1980). *The Suicide Syndrome*. London: Croom Helm.

Office of Health Economics. (1981). *Suicide and Deliberate Self-harm*. London: Office of Health Economics.

Chapter 9

British National Formulary. (1983). Drug dependence related to misuse of drugs. pp. 22–4.

Clark P., Kricka L., eds (1980). *Medical Consequences of Alcohol Abuse*. Chichester: Horwood.

Grant M., Gwinner P., eds (1979). *Alcoholism in Perspective*. London: Croom Helm.

Richter D., ed. (1979). *Addiction and Brain Damage*. London: Croom Helm.

Chapter 10

Crisp A.H. (1980). *Anorexia Nervosa: Let Me Be*. London: Academic Press.

Lipowski Z.J. (1976). Psychosomatic medicine: an overview. In: Hill O.W., ed. *Modern Trends in Psychosomatic Medicine 3*. London: Butterworth, pp. 1–20.

Palmer R.L. (1980). *Anorexia Nervosa*. Harmondsworth: Penguin Books.

Russell G.F.M. (1979). Bulimia nervosa: an ominous variant of anorexia nervosa. *Psychological Medicine*, **9**: 429–48.

Stunkard A.J. ed. (1980). *Obesity*. Philadelphia: Saunders.

Chapter 11

Bancroft J. (1974). *Deviant Sexual Behaviour: Modification and Assessment*. Oxford: Clarendon Press.

Kaplan H.S. (1974). *The New Sex Therapy*. London: Balliere Tindall.

Katchadourian H.A., Lunde D.T. (1975). *Fundamentals of Human Sexuality*. New York: Holt Rhinehart.

Kolodny R.C., Masters W.H., Johnson V.E. (1979). *Textbook of Sexual Medicine*. Boston: Little Brown.

Masters W.H., Johnson V.E. (1970). *Human Sexual Inadequacy*. London: Churchill.

Chapter 12

Bloch S., ed. (1979). *An Introduction to the Psychotherapies*. Oxford: Oxford University Press. (An excellent introductory text for all psychological methods of treatment.)

Ryle A. (1976). Group psychotherapy. *British Journal of Hospital Medicine*, **15**: 239–48.

Skynner A.C.R. (1976). Family and marital psychotherapy. *British Journal of Hospital Medicine*, **15**: 224–34.

Brandon S. (1970). Crisis theory and possibilities of therapeutic intervention. *British Journal of Psychiatry*, **117**: 627–33.

Marks I. (1976). Behavioural psychotherapy. *British Journal of Hospital Medicine*, **16**: 250–6.

Chapter 13

Cranmer J.L., Barraclough B.M., Heine B. (1982). *The Use of Drugs in Psychiatry*, 2nd ed. London: Gaskell.

Hollister L.E. (1978). *Clinical Pharmacology of Psychotherapeutic Drugs*. Edinburgh: Churchill Livingstone.

Paykel E.S., Coppen A. eds. (1979). *Psychopharmacology of Affective Disorders*. Oxford: Oxford University Press.

Silverstone T., Turner P. (1978). *Drug Treatment in Psychiatry*. London: Routledge and Kegan Paul.

Chapters 14 and 15

Gunn J., Robertson G., Dell S., Way C. (1978). *Psychiatric Aspects of Imprisonment*. London: Academic Press.

Home Office, Department of Health. (1975). *Report of the Committee on Mentally Abnormal Offenders*. London: HMSO Cmnd. 6244.

Jones K. (1972). *A History of the Mental Health Service*. London: Routledge and Kegan Paul.

Walker N. (1968). *Crime and Insanity in England*. Vol 1. Edinburgh: University Press.

Walker N., McCabe S. (1973). *Crime and Insanity in England*. Vol 2. Edinburgh: University Press.

Index